Therapeutics in Pregnancy and Lactation

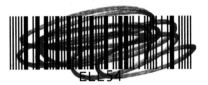

Radcliffe Medical Press

© 2000 Anne Lee, Sally Inch and David Finnigan   ✓

Radcliffe Medical Press Ltd
18 Marcham Road, Abingdon, Oxon OX14 1AA

Every effort has been made to ensure the accuracy of this text and that the best information
available has been used. This does not diminish the requirement to exercise clinical
judgement, and neither the publishers nor the authors can accept any responsibility for its use
in practice.

British Library Cataloguing in Publication Data

A catalogue record for this book is available from the British Library.

ISBN 1 85775 269 4

Typeset by Multiplex Medway Ltd, Walderslade, Kent
Printed and bound by TJ International Ltd, Padstow, Cornwall

Contents

Preface

This book has been written to assist doctors, pharmacists, midwives and other health professionals dealing with the issue of medicines use in pregnant and breastfeeding women.

The *British National Formulary* warns that 'no drug is safe beyond all doubt in early pregnancy' and that the administration of some drugs to nursing mothers may cause toxicity in the infant. Many pregnant and breastfeeding women will, nevertheless, need drug treatment and inevitably some women will become pregnant while taking medication. Decisions about the management of these women should be based on reliable information, but it is extremely difficult to obtain robust outcome data after drug exposures in pregnant or breastfeeding women. Where relevant information does exist, it may be difficult for health professionals to access it or to put it into context. This is a complex aspect of drug safety and often there are no clear answers.

In this book we have summarised the known effects of many widely used drugs and, where possible, have attempted to give guidance on the most appropriate choice of therapy in pregnant or breastfeeding women. It will provide busy health professionals with information and advice which complements that in the *British National Formulary* and other sources, helping them to ensure safe and effective drug treatment of these women.

Anne Lee
April 2000

List of contributors

Richard Ashton
Consultant Dermatologist
Royal Hospital
Haslar
Hants

Elizabeth Bardolph
Dermatology Research Nurse
Royal Hospital
Haslar
Hants

Steve Chaplin
Medical Writer
Hexham, Northumberland

Edzard Ernst
Director
Department of Complementary
    Medicine
School of Postgraduate Medicine
    and Health Sciences
University of Exeter

David Finnigan
General Practitioner
Marsden Road Health Centre
South Shields

Susanna Gilmour-White
Principal Pharmacist
South Thames Regional Drug
    Information Centre
Guy's Hospital
London

Elena Grant
Principal Pharmacist
West Midlands Regional Drug
    Information Service
Good Hope Hospital NHS Trust
Sutton Coldfield

Peter Golightly
Director
Trent Drug Information Service
Leicester Royal Infirmary

Sally Inch
Breastfeeding Advisor
Women's Centre
John Radcliffe Hospital
Oxford

Anne Lee
Principal Pharmacist
Drug Information
Glasgow Royal Infirmary

Martin Parkinson
Pharmaceutical Advisor
Dudley Health Authority

Kathryn Pughe
Senior Information Pharmacist
National Teratology Information
    Service
Drug and Therapeutics Centre
Wolfson Unit
Newcastle-upon-Tyne

Helen Seymour
Prescribing Support Manager
Drug and Therapeutics Centre
Wolfson Unit
Newcastle-upon-Tyne

Rodney Taylor
Medical Director and Consultant
   Gastroenterologist
Royal Hospital
Haslar
Hants

Simon Wills
Head of Drug Information
Drug Information Centre
St Mary's Hospital
Portsmouth

Alan James Worsley
National Teratology Information
   Service
Drug and Therapeutics Centre
Wolfson Unit
Newcastle-upon-Tyne

Phil Young
formerly: Senior Pharmacist
Prescribing Unit
Drug and Therapeutics Centre
Wolfson Unit
Newcastle-upon-Tyne

CHAPTER ONE

Principles of drug use in pregnancy

Anne Lee

Introduction

Drug use in pregnancy is an extremely difficult issue for health professionals. Since the thalidomide tragedy in the 1960s there has been increased public awareness of the risks that drug treatment can present to the developing fetus, yet most women still take medicines during pregnancy.[1,2] Many women take medicines before they know they are pregnant, and then ask whether the drug could have harmed the developing fetus. Doctors need to make decisions about which drugs to prescribe for pregnant women and which to avoid. Other health professionals, including midwives, pharmacists and health visitors, also have an important role in advising women about the potential risks of drug treatment in pregnancy.

All drugs should be avoided in pregnancy unless they are essential. In practice it may not be easy to know when drug treatment really is necessary or whether a particular medicine is an appropriate choice for a pregnant woman. This area of therapeutics, perhaps more than any other, requires a balanced approach. Being over-cautious could lead to women being denied medication of benefit or to unwarranted pregnancy termination when an exposure has already occurred. On the other hand, lack of due caution might lead to babies born harmed as a consequence of drug exposure.

The benefits of treating a pregnant woman should always be weighed against the risks of giving no medication. For example, in a woman with epilepsy it could be more hazardous not to give drug treatment, because of the risks to mother and fetus of uncontrolled seizures, than to give a drug which has the potential to cause fetal abnormality. Conversely, in a woman with acne taking long-term antibiotics, the risks associated with stopping drug treatment are minimal.

Before becoming pregnant, women may need information and advice, for example about the need to take a folic acid supplement in early pregnancy and about the possible fetal risks associated with smoking, alcohol and drugs of abuse. Health professionals need access to reliable and up-to-date information about therapeutics in pregnancy so they can give these women good advice.

Teratogenicity and drugs

The strict definition of a teratogen is an agent or factor which can cause congenital malformations. The term is now used for any agent which, given to the pregnant mother, causes or contributes to malformation or abnormal physiological function or mental development of the fetus or in the child after birth. For example, a teratogen can prevent implantation of the conceptus, cause abortion, produce intrauterine growth retardation or cause fetal death. Exposure may also have adverse effects on the neonate, or lead to functional impairment such as behavioural abnormalities or mental retardation which may not be apparent until later life.

The incidence of major malformations in the general population is estimated at between 2 and 5%, and drugs are thought to cause less than 1% of these.[3] Thus, in quantitative terms, therapeutic drugs appear not to be a significant cause of birth defects. However, most birth defects have no known cause and exposure to drugs or other teratogens may play a part in some of these. Specific birth defects are not the only consequence of exposure to a teratogen and it is possible that drugs are a factor in problems such as spontaneous miscarriage, which occurs in up to 20% of pregnancies.

Evaluation of drug safety in pregnancy

For many reasons it is extremely difficult to determine whether or not a particular agent is a teratogen.[3] Because most birth defects are rare, an increased risk posed by a teratogen may not be easily identified. Thalidomide is a potent teratogen, first-trimester exposure causing an up to 50% incidence of major malformations.[4] Most suspected teratogens, however, cause a relatively small increase in the baseline risk of malformations. For example, sodium valproate exposure increases the risk of neural tube defects by a factor of about 200, yet the overall risk of an exposed mother having a baby with spina bifida is about 1–2%.[5]

Women are generally advised to avoid medicines during pregnancy because their safety is uncertain and the study of drugs in pregnant women is usually unethical. As a result, the available data on specific drugs are often sparse and incomplete.

Epidemiological studies of drug exposure in pregnancy require large numbers of exposed infants to prove or disprove the teratogenic potential of a given drug. Most studies have inadequate statistical power because they do not include sufficient patient numbers. For example, to establish with a 95% confidence level that a drug changes the naturally occurring frequency of a congenital malformation by 1% would require a study involving about 35 000 women.[6] For this reason, no drug is safe beyond all doubt in early pregnancy.

Animal studies of reproductive toxicity are required before new drugs are licensed, but it is difficult to extrapolate the findings to human pregnancy. Drugs which produce defects in animals can be relatively safe in humans; for example, corticosteroids.[7] Of over 2000 drugs, chemicals and environmental agents shown to be teratogenic in animals, only a small number has been proven to damage the human fetus.[4]

There may be problems in distinguishing between the effect of a drug on the fetus and that of the condition for which the drug is administered. For example, debate continues about whether defects attributed to anti-epileptic drugs might be due to epilepsy itself.[8] Alternatively, a fetal disorder might produce symptoms in the mother which are treated with a drug and subsequently the drug is wrongly implicated as the cause of the disorder.

Only a few drugs (less than 50) are proven human teratogens (Table 1.1). However, no drug has proven safety based on reliable epidemiological data involving sufficient numbers of women.

Table 1.1:   Some teratogenic drugs

ACE inhibitors	Renal dysfunction and hypotension in the newborn, decreased skull ossification, hypocalvaria and renal tubular dysgenesis[9]
Alcohol	Fetal alcohol syndrome[10]
Aminoglycosides	Deafness, vestibular damage[11]
Androgens (e.g. danazol)	Masculinisation of female fetus[12]
Anti-cancer drugs	Multiple defects, abortion[13]
Anti-thyroid drugs	Fetal goitre[15]
Carbamazepine	Neural tube defects[14]
Cocaine	Cardiovascular, central nervous system defects[16]
Diethylstilboestrol	Vaginal carcinoma after *in utero* exposure[17]
Lithium	Cardiovascular defects (Ebstein's anomaly)[18]
Phenytoin	Fetal hydantoin syndrome[19]
Retinoids	Craniofacial, cardiac, central nervous system defects[20]
Sodium valproate	Neural tube defects[5]
Thalidomide	Limb-shortening defects, renal malformations, congenital heart disease[21]
Warfarin	Fetal warfarin syndrome[22]

Drugs and the fetus

The placenta is not a barrier to drugs. Nearly all drugs, except those with a very high molecular weight, such as insulin and heparin, cross the placenta to the fetus.[5] Lipid-soluble, un-ionised drugs cross more rapidly than polar drugs. In practice, virtually all drugs have the potential to affect the unborn child.

Timing of drug exposure

The effect of a drug on the developing fetus depends on several factors, including the timing of exposure, dosage, concomitant maternal disease and, in some cases, genetic susceptibility. In general, teratogens do not cause defects in all fetuses exposed at the critical period of gestation. A drug that harms a baby in one pregnancy may have no effect in a subsequent pregnancy in the same woman.

The timing of drug exposure is important in determining whether it is likely to harm the fetus. During the pre-embryonic period, which lasts until 14 days post-conception, exposure to a teratogen is believed to have an 'all or nothing' effect. Damage to all or most cells results in death of the conceptus. If only a few cells are injured, normal development is likely. Thus, women with a history of drug use in the month or so following the last menstrual period can often be reassured. Clearly, this principle only applies where the drug is completely eliminated before this time and cannot be used for drugs with a long half-life or when dates of conception are uncertain.

The fetus is most vulnerable to teratogens during the embryonic period, weeks three to eight after conception, when the major organ systems are formed. For some drugs there is a time period of highest risk for a particular defect. Exposure to sodium valproate at the time the neural tube closes (between 17 and 30 days post-conception) may result in spina bifida.[5] Cleft palate develops at about 36 days post-conception, so a drug exposure outside this period is unlikely to be implicated.

During the fetal period (week nine post-conception to birth) the fetus is less susceptible to toxic insults, although some organs, such as the cerebellum and some urogenital structures, continue to be formed. A drug given after nine weeks is more likely to cause general growth retardation or interfere with functional development within specific organ systems.[23] For example, the synthetic androgen danazol can cause virilisation of female fetuses where exposure occurs after eight weeks of gestation.[12] Warfarin may cause intracranial haemorrhage in the fetus after exposure in the second and third trimesters.[22]

Drugs taken close to term can cause predictable, pharmacological effects in the neonate. For example, non-steroidal anti-inflammatory drugs (NSAIDs) taken in the last six weeks of pregnancy can cause premature closure of the ductus arteriosus, giving rise to neonatal pulmonary hypertension.[24] Exposure to beta-blockers close to term may induce neonatal hypoglycaemia.[25] Withdrawal effects can also be a major problem in neonates born tolerant to drug effects after regular *in utero* exposure.[26]

Most drug effects will be evident at, or before, birth. However, exposure can have delayed effects, appearing years later. Diethylstilboestrol is a synthetic oestrogen which was used in the treatment of threatened spontaneous abortion. Many female fetuses exposed before the ninth week of pregnancy developed vaginal or cervical carcinoma in later life.[17,27] It has also been postulated that exposure to centrally-acting drugs might have long-term effects on neurodevelopment, but research in this area is inconclusive.[28–30]

Dose and polypharmacy

In general, teratogenicity is dose dependent. Studies have shown a significant relationship between the incidence of neural tube defects and the total daily dose, or dose per administration, of sodium valproate.[5] Animal studies have also shown that the incidence of neural tube defects correlates with high peak levels of sodium valproate.[31] However, dosage is only a relative risk factor; normal babies have been born to women who received high doses of valproate and vice versa.

There is some evidence that exposure to multiple drugs is more likely to result in abnormalities than exposure to a single drug. One study of malformations among babies born to women with epilepsy found that the incidence of birth defects increased with the number of anti-epileptics taken.[32] There was a 4% incidence of defects in babies born to women taking one drug and a 23% incidence in babies whose mothers took four or more drugs. Although this association may be partly due to confounding by disease severity this is unlikely to be the only explanation. Further evidence of such synergistic effects is lacking, but polypharmacy should be avoided where possible.

Genetic factors

There is increasing evidence, mainly from studies involving anti-epileptic drugs, that genetic factors are an important determinant of teratogenic effects.[8,33] Most anti-epileptics are converted by hepatic microsomal enzymes to epoxide intermediates which are then detoxified by epoxide hydrolase. Preliminary studies suggest that malformation rates are correlated with high levels of epoxide intermediates, particularly arene oxides.[34] Phenytoin teratogenicity can be linked with high levels of these metabolites occurring in individuals with low activity of epoxide hydrolase, the activity of which is genetically determined.[35,36] Further studies on the influence of genetic factors on teratogenicity are in progress.

The effects of pregnancy on drug handling

The physiological changes of pregnancy can affect the way the body handles drugs. Renal function increases gradually, leading to an increase in the elimination rate of drugs excreted by the kidney, such as ampicillin, gentamicin and digoxin.[37] The distribution volume may be altered because of increases in plasma volume and cardiac output. Uterine blood flow increases to 600–700 mL/min. Body water increases by about 8 litres; 60% to placenta, fetus and amniotic fluid and 40% to maternal tissues. As a result there is a decrease in the serum concentrations of many drugs, especially those with a relatively small distribution volume.[38] Protein binding of drugs also falls, partly because of a decrease in serum albumin concentrations. Consequently, the unbound (free) fraction is increased, resulting in larger distribution volumes because it is the unbound drug which is free to move into various tissue compartments. The protein binding of several anti-epileptic drugs, including phenytoin, diazepam and sodium valproate, has been shown to decrease significantly in the last trimester of pregnancy.[39]

Some drugs achieve lower serum concentrations during pregnancy. This can be important for drugs showing good correlation between plasma levels and therapeutic effect (e.g. phenytoin, lithium, carbamazepine and digoxin). Women taking these drugs should have their plasma levels monitored and dosage adjusted accordingly.

Sources of information

The problem of prescribing in pregnancy is compounded by the lack of reliable data on which to base a decision. Information about the effects of drugs in pregnancy comes mainly from case reports or epidemiological studies.[40] Case reports may signal a possible association between a drug exposure and a malformation, but many spurious or chance associations are described. Hypotheses generated from case reports must be tested by epidemiological studies. Epidemiological studies can be either case–control or cohort studies and both have important limitations. Case–control studies are usually retrospective and suffer from incompleteness and unreliability of data. Cohort studies can be either retrospective or prospective, but they have the disadvantage that very large numbers of pregnancies must be studied in order to be statistically reliable. The Boston Collaborative Perinatal Project[41] was a prospective study of more than 50 000 pregnant women exposed to about 900 drugs. Although statistically significant associations were detected in this study, no drugs were shown conclusively to be teratogenic.

Easily accessible sources of information for health professionals include the *British National Formulary (BNF)*, which contains an appendix on prescribing in pregnancy. This provides brief information on drugs which may have harmful effects in pregnancy together with the trimester of risk. However, if a drug is not listed it cannot be assumed to be safe. Manufacturers' summaries of product characteristics are another possible resource, but these are often written from a medico-legal standpoint and do not help with the decision on whether a drug is suitable for a pregnant woman. Specialised textbooks are available but can be difficult to use and expensive.[11,42]

Health professionals need a source of reliable and up-to-date information to guide them in this difficult area. All UK drug information centres can provide information and advice on drugs in pregnancy; the *BNF* gives contact details. In addition, a National Teratology Information Service provides a telephone enquiry service on all aspects of drug and chemical exposure in pregnant or potentially pregnant women. This is available free of charge to all UK health professionals. This unit has links with the National Poisons Information Service and the European Network of Teratology Information Services (ENTIS). For contact details, see the *BNF*, Appendix 4.

Some countries, including the USA and Sweden, have adopted classification systems to give an indication of the possible risks associated with the use of individual drugs during pregnancy and lactation.[43] These systems have some disadvantages, in particular safety categories allocated can differ between them. No such system is used in the UK.

Principles of drug use in pregnancy

The potential risks of drug therapy must always be considered in all women with child-bearing potential, especially as almost half of all pregnancies in the UK are unplanned. Four key questions should be asked when seeing any woman of child-bearing age:[23]

1 Is she pregnant?
2 Is she trying to become pregnant or at risk of an unplanned pregnancy?
3 Is she actively avoiding conception?
4 Can you assume she is not pregnant?

General principles of prescribing in pregnancy

- Consider non-drug treatments.
- Avoid all drugs in the first trimester if possible.
- Avoid drugs known to have harmful effects (Table 1.1). If any of these drugs must be used in a pregnant, or potentially pregnant, woman the potential risks should be discussed with her.
- Avoid new drugs. There is usually more experience with well-established preparations.
- Avoid polypharmacy.
- Use the lowest effective dose for as short a time as possible.
- Consider the need for dosing changes and therapeutic monitoring with some drugs (e.g. phenytoin, lithium).

References

1   Rubin PC, Craig GF, Gavin K *et al.* (1986) Prospective survey of use of therapeutic drugs, alcohol and cigarettes during pregnancy. *BMJ.* **292**: 81–3.

2   Rubin JD, Ferencz C, Loffredo C *et al.* (1993) Use of prescription and non-prescription drugs in pregnancy. *J Clin Epidemiol.* **46**(6): 581–9.

3   Bloomfield TH and Hawkins DF (1991) The effects of drugs on the human fetus. In *Scientific Foundations of Obstetrics and Gynaecology* (eds E Philip, M Setchell and J Ginsberg), pp. 320–36. Butterworth-Heinneman, Oxford.

4   Schardein JL (1985) *Chemically Induced Birth Defects.* Marcel Dekker, New York.

5   Omtzigt JGC, Los FJ, Grobbee DE *et al.* (1992) The risk of spina bifida aperta after first trimester valproate exposure in a prenatal cohort. *Neurology.* **42**(5): 119–25.

6   Andrews EB, Tilson HH, Hurn BAL *et al.* (1988) Acyclovir in pregnancy registry. An observational epidemiologic approach. *Am J Med.* **85**(2A): 123–8.

7   Fraser FC and Sajoo A (1995) Teratogenic potential of corticosteroids in humans. *Teratology.* **51**: 45–6.

8   Lewis DP, Van Dyke DC, Stumbo PJ *et al.* (1998) Drug and environmental factors associated with adverse pregnancy outcomes. Part 1: Anti-epileptic drugs, contraceptives, smoking, and folate. *Ann Pharmacother.* **32**: 802–17.

9   Feldcamp M, Jones KL, Ornoy A *et al.* (1997) Post-marketing surveillance for angiotensin-converting enzyme inhibitor use during pregnancy – United States, Canada and Israel 1987–1995. *JAMA.* **277**: 1193.

10 Classen SK (1981) Recognition of fetal alcohol syndrome. *JAMA.* **265**: 2436–9.

11 Briggs GG, Freeman RK, Yaffe SJ (1994) *Drugs in Pregnancy and Lactation. A reference guide to fetal and neonatal risk* (4th edn). Williams and Wilkins, Baltimore.

12 Brunskill PJ (1992) The effects of fetal exposure to danazol. *Br J Obstet Gynaecol.* **99**: 212–15.

13 Barber HRK (1981) Fetal and neonatal effects of cytotoxic agents. *Obstet Gynecol.* **58**(5): 41S–47S.

14 Rosa FW (1991) Spina bifida in infants of women treated with carbamazepine during pregnancy. *N Engl J Med.* **324**: 674–7.

15 Anon (1995) The practical management of thyroid disease in pregnancy. *Drug Ther Bull.* **33**(14): 75–7.

16 Lutiger B, Graham K, Einarson TR *et al.* (1991) Relationship between gestational cocaine use and pregnancy outcome: a meta-analysis. *Teratology.* **44**: 405–14.

17 Anon (1991) Diethylstilboestrol – effects of exposure *in utero. Drug Ther Bull.* **29**: 49–50.

18 Jacobson SJ, Jones K, Johnson K *et al.* (1992) Prospective multicentre study of pregnancy outcome after lithium exposure during first trimester. *Lancet.* **339**: 530–3.

19 Hanson JW and Smith DW (1975) The fetal hydantoin syndrome. *J Pediatr.* **87**: 285–90.

20 Lammer EJ, Hayes AM, Schunior A *et al.* (1987) Risk for major malformation among human fetuses exposed to isotretinoin (13-cis-retinoic acid). *Teratology.* **35**: 68A.

21 McBride WG (1961) Thalidomide and congenital abnormalities. *Lancet.* **2**: 1358.

22 Hall JG, Pauli RM and Wilson KM (1980) Maternal and fetal sequelae of anticoagulation during pregnancy. *Am J Med.* **68**: 122–40.

23 Anon (1996) Pre-conception, pregnancy and prescribing. *Drug Ther Bull.* **34**(4): 25–7.

24 Momma K and Takeuchi H (1983) Constriction of the fetal ductus arteriosus by non-steroidal anti-inflammatory drugs. *Prostaglandins.* **26**: 631–43.

25 Eliahou HE, Silverberg DS, Reisin E *et al.* (1978) Propranolol for the treatment of hypertension in pregnancy. *Br J Obstet Gynaecol.* **85**: 431.

26 Webster PA (1973) Withdrawal symptoms in neonates associated with maternal antidepressant therapy. *Lancet.* **2**: 318–19.

27 Giusti RM, Iwamoto K and Hatch EE (1995) Diethylstilboestrol revisited: a review of the long-term health effects. *Ann Intern Med.* **122**: 778–88.

28 Vernadakis A and Parker KK (1980) Drugs and the developing central nervous system. *Pharmacol Ther.* **11**: 593–647.

29 Viggedal G, Hagberg BS, Laegreid L *et al.* (1993) Mental development in late infancy after prenatal exposure to benzodiazepines – a prospective study. *J Child Psychol Psychiat.* **34**: 295–305.

30 Nulman I, Rovet J, Stewart DE *et al.* (1997) Neurodevelopment of children exposed *in utero* to antidepressant drugs. *N Engl J Med.* **336**: 258–62.

31 Nau H (1985) Teratogenic valproic acid concentrations: infusion by implanted minipumps vs conventional injection regimen in the mouse. *Toxicol Appl Pharmacol.* **80**: 243–50.

32 Nakane Y, Okuma T, Takahashi R *et al.* (1980) Multi-institutional study of the teratogenicity and fetal toxicity of anti-epileptic drugs: a report of a collaborative study group in Japan. *Epilepsia.* **21**: 663–80.

33 Lindhout D and Omtzigt JGC (1992) Pregnancy and the risk of teratogenicity. *Epilepsia.* **33**(4): S41–S48.

34 Lindhout D, Hoppener R and Meinardi H (1984) Teratogenicity of anti-epileptic drug combinations with special emphasis on epoxidation of carbamazepine. *Epilepsia.* **25**: 77–83.

35 Buehler BA, Delimont D, van Waes M *et al.* (1990) Prenatal prediction of the fetal hydantoin syndrome. *N Engl J Med.* **332**: 1567–72.

36 Strickler SM, Dansky LV, Miller MA *et al.* (1985) Genetic predisposition to phenytoin-induced birth defects. *Lancet.* **2**: 746–9.

37 Mucklow J (1986) The fate of drugs in pregnancy. *Clin Obstet Gynaecol.* **13**(2): 161–75.

38 Loebstein R, Lalkin A and Koren G (1997) Pharmacokinetic changes during pregnancy and their clinical relevance. *Clin Pharmacokinet.* **33**(5): 328–43.

39 Knott C and Reynolds F (1990) Therapeutic drug monitoring in pregnancy: rationale and current status. *Clin Pharmacokinet.* **19**(6): 425–33.

40 Koren G, Pastuszak A and Ito S (1998) Drugs in pregnancy. *N Eng J Med.* **338**: 1128–37.

41 Heinonen OP, Slone D and Shapiro S (1977) *Birth Defects and Drugs in Pregnancy.* Publishing Sciences Group, Acton, Massachussetts.

42 Folb PI and Graham Dukes MN (eds) (1990) *Drug Safety in Pregnancy.* Elsevier, Amsterdam.

43 Sannerstedt R, Lundborg P, Danielsson BR *et al.* (1996) Drugs during pregnancy. An issue of risk classification and information to prescribers. *Drug Safety.* **14**(2): 69–77.

CHAPTER TWO

Principles of prescribing in lactation

Elena Grant and Peter Golightly

Introduction

In the last ten years there has been a statistically significant increase in the incidence of breastfeeding in the UK.[1,2] However, the rate of decline in the first six weeks (25%) has remained unchanged. The commonest reasons given for stopping in this period are insufficient milk and sore nipples, and these can be related directly to insufficient attention being paid to teaching women the basic principles of attachment as they start to breastfeed.

The hospital practices most strongly associated with women ceasing to breastfeed include delaying the first feed, giving artificial feeds, separating mother and baby, and restricting feed frequency and duration. Although figures from surveys conducted on behalf of the UK Department of Health in 1990 and 1995 show that these practices are declining, they have probably not decreased sufficiently to have lost their negative impact on breastfeeding.

Benefits of breastfeeding

The scientific evidence supporting the beneficial effects of breastfeeding has been accumulating over several decades. The World Health Organisation (WHO) has published a *Code for Infant Feeding* to protect developing countries from being inundated with formula products which discourage breastfeeding. In such countries, infant survival often depends on breastfeeding.[3] Official recommendations that breastfeeding is preferable to use of infant formulae and that all mothers should be encouraged to breastfeed were endorsed in the

UK by the Working Party of the Panel on Child Nutrition of the Committee on Medical Aspects of Food Policy in their 1988 report.[4] In 1994, the Standing Committee on Nutrition of the British Paediatric Association published a statement summarising the current knowledge on the clinical benefits of breastfeeding in both mothers and babies.[5]

Many benefits of breastfeeding have been identified (Table 2.1). The composition of breast milk adapts to meet the changing demands of the developing infant, especially with regard to protein, fat, vitamin and mineral content. Breast milk is better digested than formula feeds due to the presence of bifidus factor. Milk is normally only produced in quantities that satisfy the nutritional requirements of the infant and which prevent overfeeding and obesity.

Table 2.1:   Benefits of breastfeeding[5]

Advantages	Comments
TO THE INFANT	

1   Reduced risk of infection:
   –   gastrointestinal infection
   –   urinary tract infection
   –   otitis media
   –   respiratory disease
   –   necrotising enterocolitis in
       pre-term neonates
	Breast milk contains secretory 1gA with specificity to antigens in the maternal gastrointestinal and respiratory tract. Other elements, e.g. lymphocytes, cytokines, and macrophages, augment this process. The protective effect of breastfeeding for more than 13 weeks remains beyond the period of breastfeeding.

2 Neurological development	Difficulties in study design have cast questions on the findings of some trials. However, well-designed trials have demonstrated a link between duration of feeding and increased scores of cognitive function.
3 Protection against later development of atopic disease	For example, there is strong evidence that the incidence of eczema is lower in breastfed infants.

4   Effects later in life:
   –   insulin-dependent
       diabetes mellitus
	A dose-dependent reduction in diabetes risk has been seen in several studies. Exposure to bovine serum albumin via infant feeding formulae may trigger the auto-immune process, leading to onset of juvenile-diabetes.

5 Sudden infant death syndrome (SIDS)	Published studies have not clearly identified a relationship between bottle feeding and SIDS, but recent findings that sleep patterns of bottle- and breastfed infants differ suggest that neurological maturation linked to dietary composition could be relevant.
TO THE MOTHER	
1 Reduction in risk of pre-menopausal breast cancer, ovarian cancer, and hip fractures	Risk of development of breast cancer before age 36 is negatively correlated with both duration of breastfeeding and number of babies breastfed.

Compared with a baby who is fully breastfed for three to four months, a bottlefed baby is:

- five times more likely to be admitted to hospital with gastroenteritis
- five times more likely to develop a urinary tract infection
- twice as likely to suffer from middle ear infection
- twice as likely to suffer from respiratory infection
- twice as likely to develop eczema or wheeze if there is a family history of atopic disease
- twice as likely to develop insulin dependent diabetes in childhood.

> **If born prematurely, the bottle-fed neonate is up to 20 times more likely to develop necrotising enterocolitis from which one in five pre-term babies will die.**

The flexibility in composition of breast milk gives a more natural balance of calcium and phosphate, leading to a very low incidence of neonatal tetany. Breast milk also presents iron in a more absorbable form than that in formula feeds. Consequently, iron-related anaemias are rare in breastfed infants. Breast milk, unlike bottle feeds, is not a means of transmission of pathogens.

The benefits of breastfeeding to the mother are largely practical and economical as well as increasing her psychological bonding to the infant. The woman who has given birth is also disadvantaged if she does not lactate. She is at increased risk of hip fracture, ovarian cancer and pre-menopausal breast cancer. One study has suggested that the relative risk of pre-menopausal breast cancer is more than doubled if parturient women bottle feed.[6] Since breast cancer affects one in 12 women in the UK, a protective effect of this magnitude is potentially very important.

Breastfeeding has an effect on fertility and this is the basis of the lactational amenorrhoea method (LAM) of contraception. Suckling causes a reduction in gonadotrophin-releasing hormone, luteinising hormone and follicle-stimulating hormone, resulting in amenorrhoea and stimulation of prolactin and milk production. The WHO has stated that LAM is an effective method of contraception offering 98% protection against pregnancy when:[7]

- a woman is fully breastfeeding (with no substitutes and at regular periods) on demand, day and night
- the baby is less than six months old
- menstruation has not returned.

Medication and breastfeeding mothers

Breastfeeding is regarded as one of the most important measures to improve child health in all societies. Health professionals should actively promote breastfeeding and facilitate its practice.

Often, literature on the use of drugs is over-cautious and may unnecessarily contraindicate the use of drugs. The content of manufacturers' data sheets are governed by the licensing regulations and a contraindication to use in breastfeeding may be based on lack of available evidence rather than known adverse effects. In current practice, greater consideration is given to the value of breastfeeding and it is necessary to appraise critically the published literature. In the absence of published data, guidance can be formulated based on a consideration of the pharmacological and pharmacokinetic properties of the drug and its side-effect profile.

The most important question to ask is whether a breastfeeding mother needs medication. If so, then a drug regimen should be chosen which will have minimal impact on the nursing infant. With careful selection it is seldom necessary to deny the infant the known benefits of breastfeeding. Only in a few instances is a temporary cessation of breastfeeding (expressing and discarding the milk) advisable (e.g. after use of a radiodiagnostic agent). In a small number of cases where a mother is on long-term medication with agents known to have potentially serious side-effects (e.g. psychotropic agents), timing of breastfeeding to avoid peak levels in milk (perhaps one to two hours after oral medication) will minimise exposure to the drug via breast milk.

Neonates and premature infants are at greater risk from exposure to drugs via breast milk because of immature excretory functions. In premature infants, the half-life may be up to five times greater than the adult value.[8] This may lead to drug accumulation and subsequent adverse effects.

Factors governing the amount of drug presented to the infant via breast milk

Accurate prediction of the extent to which a drug passes into breast milk is difficult because the process is affected by many factors whose interactions are complex and variable. In addition, there are considerable differences between individuals. Formulae for calculating the average or maximum amount of drug that an infant will ingest via breast milk have been proposed.[9,10] These are based on maternal plasma levels, the corresponding milk/plasma ratio and an assumption of the quantity of milk ingested (generally 150 mL/kg body weight per day, regardless of age). This calculated total daily dose via breast milk can be related to standard paediatric or weight-adjusted adult doses to assess the likelihood of a pharmacological or dose-related effect of the drug in the infant.

The principal determinants of the passage of drugs into breast milk are maternal factors, the characteristics of the milk and the physicochemical properties of the drug. These are outlined in Table 2.2.

Table 2.2: Factors influencing the passage of drugs into human milk[11–13]

Maternal factors	Dosage regimen
	Route of drug administration
	Drug clearance via kidneys and liver
Drug characteristics	Degree of ionisation at physiological pH
	Lipid solubility
	Protein binding
	Molecular weight
Breast physiology	Hormonal regulation of milk production
	Milk composition (particularly fat, protein and water content) and pH

Maternal factors

In general, there is a direct relationship between maternal dose and subsequent milk levels. The route of drug administration will affect maternal plasma levels. Parenteral drug administration will normally produce higher plasma levels than drugs taken orally. Drugs given by inhalation or topically normally give only very low systemic levels. Dose frequency will affect the times of peak concentrations in plasma and milk and the ability to time breastfeeding to avoid maximum concentrations in milk in the few cases where this is necessary.

The mother's ability to excrete the drug will also influence milk levels of the drug. Accumulation due to renal or hepatic impairment may pose an increased hazard to the infant.

Drug characteristics

The main characteristics of the drug which influence its passage into breast milk are the degree of ionisation (pKa value), the protein binding capacity, lipid solubility and molecular weight.

There is a pH gradient between plasma (7.4) and breast milk (6.9). In general, milk levels of basic drugs will be higher than those of acidic drugs. This is seen in practice as weak acids such as penicillins, aspirin, sulphonamides, diuretics and barbiturates are present in milk at levels less than half of the corresponding maternal plasma level (milk/plasma ratio <0.5). Conversely, weak bases such as erythromycin, histamine H_2 antagonists and isoniazid have a milk/plasma ratio of >1. These drugs may have milk levels which are many times greater than maternal plasma levels. However, this is not to imply that basic drugs will be associated with toxicity in the infant as total amounts of drug ingested are still generally low and other factors, such as protein binding, will influence excretion into milk.

Drugs which are highly protein bound in maternal plasma have a lower potential to achieve high breast milk levels, irrespective of their pKa value. Warfarin is 95% protein bound in maternal plasma and appears in breast milk in only very small quantities.

The partition coefficient of a drug is a measure of its lipid solubility. Breast milk may be regarded as a fat-in-water emulsion. Drugs with low lipid solubility, even though they may be weak bases with low protein binding, will not achieve significant levels in breast milk as they cannot penetrate lipid barriers. Since the lipid content of breast milk varies, some variations in drug levels may be seen at different stages of lactation.

The molecular weight of a drug is a limited but significant determinant of drug excretion into breast milk. Drugs with a molecular weight of less than about 200 (e.g. alcohol and lithium salts) appear in breast milk very rapidly after maternal ingestion. It is likely that these small molecules pass into breast milk largely independently of the factors outlined above. They may pass through intercellular clefts, bypassing multiple cellular lipid barriers between serum and milk.

Breast physiology

The volume of milk and yield capacity of each breast may have minor influences on the amount of drug ingested by the infant. These factors often show considerable variation between and within individuals.

Infant factors

The age of the infant is important in calculating the potential risk of adverse reactions. In premature or newborn infants, renal and hepatic functions are not fully developed and there is a risk of drug accumulation. Usually, renal and hepatic functions mature within two to four weeks after birth. Older infants will ingest decreasing amounts of drug as they are weaned from breast milk on to solid foods.

Drug exposure depends not only on the volume of milk ingested but also on the extent of absorption from the gastrointestinal tract. Some drugs normally given by injection are destroyed in the gut (e.g insulin and heparin). Since the infant receives these by the oral route, they do not pass into the systemic circulation and thus pose no hazard.

The infant's tissue receptor sensitivity may also influence the risk of adverse drug reactions. A few drugs may cause idiosyncratic or allergic reactions unrelated to the amount ingested.

Drug safety profile

The intrinsic toxicity of a drug is a major factor to be considered when assessing whether a mother on medication may safely breastfeed. A check on whether the drug is licensed for use in infants may give some guidance on this question. The side-effect profile of the drug will indicate potential hazards to the infant. Adverse reactions may be either dose related or idiosyncratic.

Drugs with long half-lives or with active metabolites may prolong exposure to the drug in milk and increase the risk of an adverse reaction in the infant. As a general rule, exposure to such agents in breast milk should be avoided, particularly in premature or newborn infants where immature excretory functions may further prolong exposure.

Classification of maternal drug therapy

By combining theoretical considerations and practical experience, maternal therapy may be classified according to the degree of risk it poses to the breastfed infant. Real effects are those demonstrated to have occurred in clinical practice. Possible effects are those which might be anticipated by extrapolating from pharmacological and adverse effects encountered in the clinical use of a drug in a paediatric population.

In terms of safety, a drug may be classified into three categories:

1 **unsuitable for use in breastfeeding mothers**. This category is where the risk (known or theoretical) outweighs the benefits of breastfeeding. Drugs in this category include those with high intrinsic toxicity, e.g antineoplastic agents, and those where serious effects have been documented, e.g lithium and high-dose oestrogens. In practice, the number of reports of serious effects is very small. Drugs in this category are listed in Table 2.3.
2 **drugs to be used with caution and only when mother and infant can be adequately monitored**. For drugs in this category, a clinical decision is normally needed for each specific case. Although published data and long-term clinical experience can assist in this process, it is difficult to formulate general rules. Examples of drugs in this category are those causing minor effects in the infant, e.g. drowsiness with antihistamines, or those where minor effects may be anticipated

on theoretical grounds, e.g. propylthiouracil, and those for which insufficient data are available to permit classification as safe, e.g. new drugs, IV metronidazole.

3   **drugs which appear safe in breastfeeding**. Here, risks are so small or non-existent and are clearly outweighed by the benefits of breastfeeding. Drugs are assigned to this category because they are not excreted into milk, not absorbed from the infant's gut, they have low intrinsic toxicity or are present in milk in such small amounts that they pose no hazard.

Table 2.3:   Some drugs contraindicated in breastfeeding

Drug	Comments
Amiodarone	Theoretical risk of thyroid disturbance because of high iodine content
Antineoplastic agents	Theoretical risk of blood dyscrasias
Chloramphenicol	Theoretical risk of blood dyscrasias
Dapsone	Haemolytic anaemia reported
Doxepin	Case report of profound respiratory depression on 75 mg daily
Ergotamine	Risk of ergotism in infants
Gold salts	Risk of hypersensitivity reactions and of haematological and renal toxicity
Iodides (including some cough preparations)	Theoretical risk of thyroid disturbance
Indomethacin	Case of infant convulsions reported
Lithium	Tremor and involuntary movements reported
Oestrogens (high dose)	May cause feminisation of male infants
Phenindione	Case of haematoma and abnormal blood coagulation reported
Radioisotopes	Radiation exposure
Vitamin D (high dose)	Case report of hypercalcaemia in infant

Drugs with an adverse effect on lactation

Only a few drugs are known to affect lactation adversely. Oestrogens, particularly in high dose, may decrease milk production and the Family Planning Association recommends that oestrogen-containing oral contraceptives should be avoided. The progestogen-only oral contraceptive does not adversely influence milk production.[13]

Drugs to enhance or suppress lactation

The dopamine receptor agonists bromocriptine and cabergoline are licensed in the UK for suppression of lactation. However, they are not recommended for routine suppression or relief of symptoms of post-partum pain and engorgement which can be adequately treated with simple analgesics and breast support.[14] High-dose oestrogens are no longer used to suppress lactation because of their association with thromboembolism.

There are no preparations which currently have a UK licence for stimulation of lactation. Metoclopramide (a dopamine D2 antagonist), by acting on dopamine receptors in the pituitary, causes an increase in prolactin secretion and studies conducted in the 1980s showed that milk production was improved in women up to three to four months post-partum.[15-17] Only short-term benefits were seen and repeat courses were often required to maintain successful lactation. The drug has been used in an attempt to benefit early and late lactational failure and to maintain milk supplies by expression in women delivering prematurely. Two drugs with similar modes of action to metoclopramide – domperidone and sulpiride – have been shown to improve milk yield in women with inadequate lactation.[18-20]

Guidelines for prescribing for breastfeeding mothers

The following principles should be followed when prescribing for breastfeeding mothers:

- Unnecessary drug use should be avoided and use of over-the-counter (OTC) products limited. Breastfeeding mothers should seek advice on the suitability of OTC products.
- The benefit/risk ratio should be assessed for both mother and infant.
- Use of drugs known to cause serious toxicity in adults or children should be avoided.
- Drugs licensed for use in infants do not generally pose a hazard.
- Neonates (and particularly premature infants) are at greater risk from exposure to drugs via breast milk because of immature excretory functions and the consequent risk of drug cumulation.
- A regimen and route of administration which presents the minimum amount of drug to the infant should be chosen.
- Long-acting formulations of drugs likely to cause serious side-effects (e.g. antipsychotic agents) are best avoided as it is difficult to time feeds to avoid significant amounts of drug in breast milk.
- Multiple drug regimes may pose an increased risk, especially when adverse effects such as drowsiness are additive.
- Infants exposed to drugs via breast milk should be monitored for unusual signs or symptoms.
- New drugs, for which little data are available, are best avoided.

References

1   White A, Freeth S and O'Brien M (1992) *Infant Feeding 1990. A survey carried out by the Social Survey Department of OPCS on behalf of the Department of Health, the Scottish Home and Health Department, the Welsh Office and the Department of Health and Social Services in Northern Ireland.* HMSO, London.

2   Office for National Statistics (1997) Breastfeeding in the United Kingdom in 1995. In: *Infant Feeding 1995.* ONS, London.

3   World Health Organisation (1991) *Contemporary Patterns of Breastfeeding. Report on the WHO Collaborative Study on Breastfeeding.* WHO, Geneva.

4   Department of Health and Social Security Committee on Medical Aspects of Food Policy (1988) *Present Day Practice in Infant Feeding: third report.* Report on Health and Social Subjects No. 32. HMSO, London.

5   Standing Committee on Nutrition of the British Paediatric Association (1994) Is breastfeeding beneficial in the UK? *Arch Dis Child.* **71**: 376–80.

6   Heinig MJ and Dewey KG (1997) Health effects of breastfeeding for mothers: a critical review. *Nutrition Research Review.* **10**: 35–56.

7   Belfield T (1999) *Family Planning Association Contraceptive Handbook. A guide for family planning and other health professionals* (3rd edn). FPA, London.

8   Haraldsson A and Geven W (1989) Half-life of maternal labetalol in a premature infant. *Pharm Weekbl (Sci).* **11**: 229–31.

9   Atkinson HC and Bigg EJ (1990) Prediction of drug distribution into human milk from physicochemical characteristics. *Clin Pharmacokinet.* **18**(2): 151–67.

10 Wilson JT, Brown RD, Chere KD *et al.* (1980) Drug excretion in human breast milk: principles, pharmacokinetics and projected consequences. *Clin Pharmacokinet.* **5**: 1–66.

11 Bennett PN (1996) *Drugs and Human Lactation* (2nd edn). Elsevier, Amsterdam.

12 Lawrence RA (1994) *Breastfeeding. A guide for the medical profession* (4th edn). CV Mosby Company, St Louis.

13 Anderson PO (1991) Drug use during breastfeeding. *Clin Pharm.* **10**: 594–624.

14 *British National Formulary No. 38 (Sept)* (1999) Royal Pharmaceutical Society of Great Britain/British Medical Association.

15 Kauppila A, Kivinen S, Ylikorkala O *et al.* (1981) A dose-response relation between improved lactation and metoclopramide. *Lancet.* **1**: 1175–7.

16 Ehrenkranz RA and Ackermin BA (1986) Metoclopramide effect on faltering milk production by mothers of premature infants. *Paediatrics.* **78**: 614–20.

17 Lewis PJ, Devenish C, Kahn C *et al.* (1980) Controlled trial of metoclopramide and the initiation of breastfeeding. *Br J Clin Pharmacol.* **9**: 217–19.

18 Petroglia F, De Leo V, Satdelli S *et al.* (1985) Domperidone in defective and insufficient lactation. *Eur J Obstet Gynecol Reprod Biol.* **19**: 281–7.

19 Aono T, Aki T, Koike K *et al.* (1982) Effect of sulpiride on poor puerperal lactation. *Am J Obstet Gynecol.* **143**: 927–32.

20 Ylikorkala O, Kauppila A, Krvinen S *et al.* (1982) Sulpiride improves inadequate lactation. *BMJ Clin Res Ed.* **285**: 249–51.

CHAPTER THREE

Common problems in pregnancy

Anne Lee

Most women will experience troublesome pregnancy-related symptoms at some stage and, in general, will seek professional advice before taking any medicine. Although drug treatment is often unnecessary, there are many situations where symptom relief will benefit the mother without detrimental effects on the fetus. Common problems include nausea and vomiting, heartburn, constipation, haemorrhoids, vaginitis, leg cramps, migraine, threadworm and scabies.

Nausea and vomiting

Nausea and vomiting are the most frequent and troublesome symptoms of early pregnancy, affecting up to 70% of women.[1] Many women consider this a normal part of pregnancy and do not seek medical advice. The causes of these symptoms are still uncertain, although human chorionic gonadotrophin (HCG) and raised thyroxine levels or suppressed thyroid-stimulating hormone (TSH) levels have been implicated.[1] Although commonly referred to as 'morning sickness', symptoms can occur at any time of day or night. Nausea and vomiting usually begin shortly after the first missed menstrual period and tend to resolve by 12 to 16 weeks gestation. There is no evidence of an adverse effect on fetal outcome; pregnancies associated with mild to moderate nausea and vomiting are less likely to end in miscarriage, pre-term delivery or stillbirth, and show no increase in the risk of congenital malformations.[1] These symptoms can generally be managed without drug treatment. Women with morning symptoms may find that eating a biscuit or dry toast before getting out of bed helps. Eating small carbohydrate-containing snacks like crackers or toast throughout the day may prevent or relieve symptoms, although the effectiveness of these measures has not been studied.[2] Drinking regular, small amounts of water or other fluid and resting can also be helpful. Non-drug treatments which may be effective in some women include acupressure at the Neiguan (P6) point in the wrist, or ginger. A review of studies examining the efficacy of acupressure has demonstrated its efficacy in the treatment of non-pregnancy-related emesis.[3] Of six studies involving pregnant women, all of which were of crossover design or included a control group, only one found no evidence of efficacy.[4] These results are encouraging and there is no reason to believe that properly applied pressure at this particular acupressure point would be harmful. This intervention may be recommended to women who are troubled by nausea and vomiting (wristbands commercially available for travel sickness can be tried).

Although ginger is a widely recommended treatment, the published data are too limited to support its use, although it is unlikely to be harmful.[4]

In some pregnancies vomiting becomes severe and intractable (hyperemesis gravidarum). About 0.5 to 10 per thousand pregnancies are affected.[5] Persistent vomiting and severe nausea progress to hyperemesis if a woman is unable to maintain adequate hydration, and fluid and electrolyte status are jeopardised. There may also be evidence of body weight loss, muscle wasting, ptyalism or spitting. Onset of symptoms occurs in the first trimester, usually in weeks six to eight. Persistent vomiting throughout pregnancy and particularly in the third trimester suggests intercurrent disease.[6] Women with a diagnosis of hyperemesis should have an ultrasound scan of the uterus to confirm gestational age and to diagnose multiple pregnancy and exclude hydatidiform mole, both of which are associated with an increased incidence of hyperemesis.[1] Management should include hospitalisation, intravenous fluid and electrolyte replacement, thiamine (vitamin B_1) supplementation, use of conventional anti-emetics and psychological support. If a woman presents with persistent, severe vomiting, it is reasonable for the GP to prescribe an antihistamine anti-emetic. Specialist advice should be sought if there is no improvement within 24 to 48 hours.

Doctors may be reluctant to prescribe anti-emetics, even when vomiting is severe, due to fears of teratogenicity, but for some agents there is a large body of data showing no evidence of such effect. Debendox (an anti-emetic containing the antihistamine doxylamine, dicyclomine and pyridoxine) was widely used in pregnancy, having been taken by over 30 million women worldwide. However, it was withdrawn from the market in 1983 as a result of litigation claiming that it had caused congenital malformations. Several large studies found no evidence that the preparation is teratogenic.[7,8] Ironically, there are more safety data for this than any other anti-emetic.

There are few comparative safety or efficacy data on which to base drug selection. In general, it seems logical to choose an agent with which there is considerable experience. On this basis, antihistamine anti-emetics, such as promethazine and cyclizine, are the drugs of choice as they have been widely used without evidence of adverse fetal effects.[9,10] A meta-analysis of 24 studies including more than 200 000 women exposed to antihistamines, used mainly for first-trimester nausea and vomiting, concluded that there was no increased teratogenic risk.[11] Promethazine may be given orally or by IM injection; for oral administration the theoclate salt is longer acting. A systematic review of the effectiveness of interventions for nausea and vomiting in early pregnancy confirms that there is clear evidence of efficacy for antihistamine anti-emetics.[12]

The phenothiazine anti-emetic prochlorperazine is very widely used during pregnancy in the UK. The frequency of congenital malformations was no greater than expected among the children of 877 women exposed during the first trimester.[9] Three other studies of exposure in early pregnancy found no evidence of an increased risk of malformation.[13] The availability of a rectal preparation is an advantage.

Metoclopramide and domperidone are generally considered safe for use in pregnancy, although they are used less often than antihistamine or phenothiazine anti-emetics and evidence from controlled studies is lacking.[13,14] Metoclopramide is associated with an increased risk of extrapyramidal reactions in young women, so it is best reserved for use when first-line agents have been ineffective.

Pyridoxine (vitamin B_6) has been investigated in two randomised controlled trials (in a dose of 25 mg three times a day[15] or 30 mg daily.[16] In the first of these there was no significant improvement in vomiting and in the second there was significant improvement only in women with severe symptoms.

There are anecdotal reports of efficacy with the 5-HT$_3$ antagonist ondansetron in intractable hyperemesis.[17,18] However, it was no more effective than promethazine in a small comparative study.[19] Evidence of safety and efficacy is insufficient to support the use of this drug.

There is now a reasonable amount of evidence supporting the efficacy of corticosteroids in hyperemesis. Recent uncontrolled studies have noted a dramatic response to oral prednisolone or IV hydrocortisone in women with persistent nausea and vomiting despite adequate IV fluid replacement, thiamine supplements and regular anti-emetics.[20–22] Randomised controlled trials of this therapy are now underway.

Table 3.1:   Anti-emetics

Class	Agents	Comments
Recommended		
Antihistamines	• Cyclizine 50 mg up to tid • Promethazine theoclate 25 mg at bedtime, increased if necessary to 100 mg daily	• **First choice** • No evidence of increased risk to fetus
Phenothiazines	• Prochlorperazine 20 mg orally or 25 mg by suppository initially, then 5–10 mg orally two to three times daily	• **Second choice**
	• Chlorpromazine	• May be used occasionally in resistant hyperemesis
Use with caution		
Dopamine antagonists	• Metoclopramide 10 mg tid (5 mg in women 15–19 yrs under 60 kg)	• **Third choice**
	• Domperidone (oral) 10–20 mg every 4–8 hours (rectal) 30–60 mg every 4–8 hours	
Avoid		
5HT$_3$ antagonists	• Ondansetron • Granisetron • Tropisetron	• Safety in pregnancy not established

Pain

Minor aches and pains often do not require drug treatment, especially in the first trimester. However, simple analgesics may be needed for headache or musculoskeletal or dental pain. In the UK, analgesics are the drugs taken most frequently by pregnant women.[23]

Paracetamol is the analgesic of choice in pregnancy. It has been used routinely during all stages of pregnancy for pyrexia and pain relief, without evidence of harmful effects on the fetus.[9,10] Aspirin has also been widely used throughout pregnancy. Overall, there is no evidence that its use is associated with an increased risk of birth defects.[13] Exposure in late pregnancy, however, can cause haemorrhage, and may prolong, or delay the onset of, labour and cause increased blood loss.[24] There is also a risk of closure of the ductus arteriosus *in utero*. High-dose aspirin, or chronic use of therapeutic doses, should be avoided throughout pregnancy and particularly in the third trimester. The thromboxane antagonist properties of low-dose aspirin (60 mg daily) have been studied in the prevention of pre-eclampsia in at-risk women; a study involving more than 9000 women suggested that aspirin had no adverse effects on the fetus.[25]

Non-steroidal anti-inflammatory agents (NSAIDs) should be avoided if possible in early pregnancy due to the lack of data on their effects. In late pregnancy they have the potential to cause premature closure of the ductus arteriosus; the risk of this complication is greater with high doses, with high-potency drugs such as indomethacin and with exposure after 32 weeks gestation (*see also* Chapter 12).[26,27]

Despite the lack of data on the safety of NSAIDs in pregnancy, none have been shown to increase the risk of birth defects, although a possible association with gastroschisis (a congenital defect in which loops of intestine protrude through the abdominal wall) has been suggested.[28] Women who have taken NSAIDs inadvertently in pregnancy can be reassured that the risks to the fetus are minimal. Although topical NSAIDs may have fewer systemic effects than oral medication, these effects can occur, so these products should be used with caution in pregnant women.

Opioid analgesics have the potential to cause dependence and withdrawal symptoms in the neonate if used or abused regularly during pregnancy.[29,30] Although some epidemiological studies have suggested an association between opioids and specific congenital malformations, overall there is no good evidence that the use of therapeutic doses in pregnancy has an adverse effect on fetal development.[13,31] Opioids may be used at any stage of pregnancy for the short-term treatment of moderate to severe pain. There is more experience with codeine than with other agents.

Table 3.2:   Analgesics in pregnancy

Class	Agents	Comments
Recommended		
Non-opioid analgesics	• Paracetamol	• **First choice**
		• Avoid high doses or prolonged exposure
Opioid analgesics	• Codeine	• No evidence of increased risk to fetus
	• Dihydrocodeine	• No evidence of increased risk to fetus
	• Morphine	• Treatment of choice for severe pain
	• Methadone	• May be used in pregnancy for opioid dependence

Table 3.2: continued

Class	Agents	Comments
Compound analgesics	• co-codamol	• No evidence of increased risk to fetus
	• co-dydramol	• No evidence of increased risk to fetus
	• co-proxamol	
Use with caution		
Non-opioid analgesics	• Aspirin	• Avoid in late pregnancy; Potential to delay or prolong labour; impaired platelet function and risk of haemorrhage
	• Benorylate	• As above
	• Nefopam	• Limited experience in pregnancy
Opioid analgesics	• Tramadol	• Limited experience in pregnancy
Compound analgesics	• co-codaprin	
Opioid agonist/antagonists	• Buprenorphine	• Limited experience in pregnancy
	• Pentazocine	• Limited experience in pregnancy
NSAIDs		• Limited experience in pregnancy
	• Ibuprofen	• NSAID of choice where one is indicated

Heartburn

Heartburn affects as many as 70% of pregnant women; it can occur at any stage but is most common in the third trimester.[32] Precipitating factors include posture, especially stooping or lying down, and eating. Simple measures such as avoiding 'trigger' foods, not eating close to bedtime, sleeping with extra pillows, and trying to avoid stooping may help relieve symptoms.[33] Antacids may be prescribed; they have been widely prescribed at all stages of pregnancy without evidence of adverse effects. There is no evidence that one antacid is superior to others although palatability is important. Aluminium hydroxide or magnesium trisilicate (both available as chewable tablets or mixture) are cheap and may be useful. Preparations containing aluminium may worsen constipation where this is a problem. Co-magaldrox (a mixture of aluminium hydroxide and magnesium hydroxide) may be prescribed as tablet or suspension. This preparation is relatively inexpensive and has a low sodium content. Alginate-containing preparations are generally more expensive and there is no evidence that they are more effective.

It has been suggested that heartburn is sometimes due to reflux of alkali from lower down the gastrointestinal tract back into the stomach. If antacids are ineffective, very dilute acids may be effective in some women. A solution of hydrochloric acid (0.1 ml diluted in 10 ml flavoured syrup) has been used, but no commercial preparation is available. Lemon juice or acidic lemonade may be more palatable alternatives.[33]

Histamine (H_2) receptor antagonists, such as cimetidine, and proton pump inhibitors, such as omeprazole, should not be used for symptomatic relief of heartburn because their safety in pregnancy has not been established (*see* Chapter 4).

Table 3.3:   Antacids and other agents to treat heartburn

Class of drug	Agents	Comments
Recommended		
Aluminium-containing preparations	• Aluminium hydroxide	• May cause constipation
Magnesium-containing preparations	• Magnesium trisilicate or carbonate	• Avoid if sodium intake is important
	• Magnesium hydroxide	
Preparations containing dimethicone		• No clear advantages over simple antacids
Preparations containing alginates	• Algicon, Gaviscon, Gastrocote	• No clear advantages over simple antacids
Dilute acid preparations	• Hydrochloric acid 0.1 ml in 10 ml	• May be effective in some women
Avoid		
Preparations containing bismuth		• Bismuth is potentially neurotoxic
Sodium bicarbonate		• May cause metabolic disturbance
H_2-receptor antagonists	• Cimetidine • Ranitidine • Famotidine • Nizatidine	• Safety in pregnancy is not established
Proton pump inhibitors	• Omeprazole • Lansoprazole • Pantoprazole • Rabeprazole	• Safety in pregnancy is not established

Constipation

Constipation is common, especially in later pregnancy, as a consequence of reduced gastrointestinal motility and increased levels of circulating progesterone. Women normally troubled by constipation often find the problem worsens in pregnancy. Increasing dietary fibre with bran or wheat fibre, fluid intake and exercise should bring relief in many cases.[34] Medication which may cause or exacerbate the problem, such as iron preparations or aluminium-containing antacids, should be stopped if possible.

Laxatives should be given only after these approaches have failed.[33] Bulk-forming agents, including bran, ispaghula and sterculia, should be tried first. Docusate sodium, which acts as a stimulant and a softening agent, and lactulose have been used in pregnancy with no evidence of adverse effects. These are useful second-line agents. Stimulant laxatives, such as bisacodyl and senna, are systemically absorbed and so best avoided in pregnancy.[33] In theory, they may cause uterine contractions if used in the third trimester. If other treatments have been ineffective, senna may be used short term.

Saline laxatives, such as magnesium and sodium salts, should be avoided in pregnancy as they may cause electrolyte disturbances. Lubricant preparations, such as liquid paraffin, are also best avoided due to their potential to cause adverse effects such as aspiration pneumonitis.[35] If persistent constipation is not treated, haemorrhoids may develop.

Table 3.4: Laxatives

Class of drug	Agents	Comments
Recommended		
Bulk-forming agents	• Bran • Ispaghula husk • Sterculia	• **First choice**
Osmotic laxatives	• Lactulose	• No evidence of adverse effects
Stimulant laxatives	• Bisacodyl • Senna	• May be considered where other agents have been ineffective • May cause uterine contractions if used in the third trimester
Other		
	• Docusate sodium • Magnesium salts	• No evidence of adverse effects • May cause electrolyte disturbances
Avoid		
Faecal softeners	• Liquid paraffin	
Stimulant laxatives	• Danthron	• Contraindicated due to carcinogenicity in rodents

Haemorrhoids

Haemorrhoids commonly occur for the first time during pregnancy. Constipation tends to worsen the condition and should be treated if present (*see* above).[33] Topical preparations can be recommended for symptomatic relief if necessary (*see British National Formulary* 1.7.1). If the haemorrhoids are swollen and painful the application of a cold compress or ice pack, such as a pack of frozen peas, may bring relief. Women may be advised that haemorrhoids usually resolve spontaneously after delivery.

Candidiasis

Vaginal candidiasis (thrush) is a frequent problem in pregnancy and occurs up to ten times as often as in non-pregnant women. It can be difficult to eradicate during pregnancy but usually clears spontaneously after delivery. Typical symptoms are vaginal discharge and pruritus. Rarely, congenital candida infection can affect infants of very low birth weight and manifest with pneumonia and skin reactions.[33] Candida infection should be treated with a topical imidazole anti-fungal. Pessaries may be supplemented with cream for vulval irritation if required. Although there is no evidence that other anti-fungals have harmful effects in human pregnancy, some of the newer agents have shown toxic effects in animal studies and should be avoided.[36]

Table 3.5: Vaginal candidiasis

Class	Agent	Comments
Recommended		
Imidazoles (local): All available as cream and vaginal tablet	• Clotrimazole • Econazole • Isoconazole • Miconazole	• **First choice**
Avoid		
Polyenes	• Nystatin	• Less effective than local imidazoles
Imidazoles (systemic)	• Itraconazole • Fluconazole	• Limited experience in pregnancy

Trichomoniasis

The protozoan *Trichomonas vaginalis* is frequently isolated from vaginal secretions during pregnancy. It is often associated with other sexually transmitted diseases so these should be sought when the organism is identified. Trichomonas infection may cause severe symptomatic vaginitis in some women, although up to 50% of those carrying the organism are asymptomatic. Vaginal discharge is the most common complaint although the classically described green, frothy discharge is uncommon.[33] Metronidazole is highly effective in trichomonas infection; a seven-day course of 200 mg three times daily or 400 mg twice a day is usually effective. Although this drug has been shown to be carcinogenic in rodents and mutagenic in bacteria, there is no evidence of teratogenicity in humans. Recent studies have shown that the incidence of malformations in babies born to women who have taken metronidazole in early pregnancy is no higher that that in the general population.[37–39]

Leg cramps

Painful cramps in the calf muscles are common in pregnancy, especially in the third trimester; the cause is unknown. A systematic review of published data concludes that there is no evidence of benefit for calcium supplements and inadequate evidence of benefit for sodium chloride (based on a single study).[40] The only treatment strategy that can be recommended is stretching or massaging the affected muscle during the attack. Quinine salts should not be used in pregnancy because of their stimulant effects on the uterus which could lead to spontaneous abortion or premature labour.

Restless legs syndrome

Restless legs syndrome may occur during pregnancy. It is an uncomfortable condition commonly described as creeping or crawling sensations deep within the legs which may be relieved by walking. Patients should be advised that symptoms remit after delivery. The condition may be associated with underlying anaemia; if this is corrected the symptoms usually remit.

Cough and cold remedies

Many preparations for colds contain a sympathomimetic decongestant such as pseudoephedrine or phenylpropanolamine, or an antihistamine such as brompheniramine, possibly in combination with an analgesic and/or expectorant. There is no evidence that any of these preparations is harmful in pregnancy.[9,10,13] However, as their efficacy is questionable, they are best avoided in pregnancy. Women should be advised to avoid combination products and to take paracetamol for symptom relief. For nasal congestion, menthol inhalations may be helpful.

Similarly, there is a lack of data on the safety of commonly used cough medicines in pregnancy but these preparations are also of limited benefit. Opioid cough suppressants are best avoided, although short-term use is unlikely to present a risk to the fetus. There is no reason to believe that expectorants or demulcents are harmful, but they are of limited efficacy. Cough and throat lozenges are unlikely to have systemic effects and can be recommended.

Migraine

Migraine often improves during pregnancy, particularly in the second and third trimesters. If attacks occur during pregnancy, non-drug treatments such as relaxation, sleep and massage should be tried first.[41] If drug treatment is required, paracetamol is the preferred analgesic, although ibuprofen may also be used. Anti-emetics such as buclizine, cyclizine, prochlorperazine or metoclopramide (the latter has the additional benefit of reducing gastric statis and improving delivery of analgesics) may also be given (*see* Nausea and vomiting, p. 23). The 5-HT$_1$ agonists (sumatriptan and related drugs) should be avoided. There is little information about their effects on the fetus, although a recent prospective outcome study found no evidence of an increased risk of major defects.[42]

Prophylactic treatment is rarely indicated during pregnancy and should be reserved for women with long-lasting or frequent attacks where standard treatment approaches are not sufficiently effective.[41] Prophylaxis should not be used in the first trimester as there is inadequate evidence of safety; in later stages, a beta-blocker or pizotifen are possible options.

Threadworms

Threadworm infestation is common in pregnancy. Women should be advised to try and eradicate infection through rigorous measures of hygiene, which will break the life cycle of the *Enterobius* parasite. With daily changing of bedlinen and nightwear, thorough scrubbing of hands and nails after going to the toilet and avoiding scratching the perianal area, the problem should clear up within a week or two. None of the available threadworm treatments have been proven safe in pregnancy and drug treatment is best avoided, particularly in the first trimester.[43] Mebendazole is poorly absorbed from the gut so is unlikely to present a risk to the fetus, although toxicity in animal studies has been noted. Outwith the first trimester, mebendazole may be used if treatment is considered necessary.[44,45] There is no evidence that piperazine exposure is harmful; women exposed inadvertently should be reassured.

Scabies and headlice

There is a lack of data on the effects of headlice and scabies treatments on the fetus. Malathion, an organophosphorous insecticide, is poorly absorbed from the skin. There is no evidence that use at recommended doses is harmful, although published information is limited.[46] Similarly, little is known about the potential risks of the pyrethroids (permethrin and phenothrin) which are now in widespread use for these indications.[47] Of these agents, malathion is first choice in pregnancy. Aqueous preparations are preferable to the alcoholic lotions. If either malathion or pyrethroids are used, women should be advised not to exceed the recommended dose and that they should not be used repeatedly. Headlice should be managed without recourse to topical treatment if possible.

References

1   Nelson-Piercy C (1998) Treatment of nausea and vomiting in pregnancy: when should it be treated and what can be safely taken? *Drug Safety.* **19**(2): 155–64.

2   Chapter 3 (1995) Unpleasant symptoms in pregnancy. In *A Guide to Effective Care in Pregnancy and Childbirth* (2nd edn) (eds M Enkin, MJNC Keirse, M Renfrew *et al.*) Oxford University Press, Oxford.

3   Vickers AJ (1996) Can acupuncture have specific effects on health? A systematic review of acupuncture in anti-emesis trials. *J Roy Soc Med.* **89**: 303–11.

4   Aikins Murphy P (1998) Alternative therapies for nausea and vomiting of pregnancy. *Obstet Gynecol.* **91**: 149–55.

5   Hod M, Orvieto R, Kaplan B *et al.* (1994) Hyperemesis gravidarum: a review. *J Reprod Med.* **39**: 605–12.

6   Fagan EA (1996) Disorders of the gastrointestinal tract. In *Medical Disorders in Obstetric Practice* (3rd edn). Blackwell Science, Oxford.

7   Fleming DM, Knox JDE and Crombie DL (1981) Debendox in early pregnancy and fetal malformation. *BMJ.* **283**: 99.

8   McCredie J, Kricker A, Elliott J *et al.* (1984) The innocent bystander. Doxylamine/ dicyclomine/pyridoxine and congenital limb defects. *Med J Aust.* **140**: 525.

9   Heinonen OP, Slone D and Shapiro S (1977) *Birth Defects and Drugs in Pregnancy.* John-Wright PSG, Littleton, Massachussetts.

10 Aselton P, Jick H, Milunsky A *et al.* (1985) First trimester drug use and congenital disorders. *Obstet Gynecol.* **65**: 451–5.

11 Seto A, Einarson T and Koren G (1997) Pregnancy outcome following first-trimester exposure to antihistamines – meta-analysis. *Am J Perinatol.* **14**: 119–24.

12 Jewell DJ and Young G (1999) Interventions for nausea and vomiting in early pregnancy (Cochrane review). In *The Cochrane Library*, Issue 1. Update Software, Oxford.

13 Friedman JM and Polifka JE (1996) *The Effects of Drugs on the Fetus and Nursing Infant. A handbook for health care professionals.* John Hopkins University Press, Baltimore.

14 Domperidone monograph in Reprotox, Reprorisk (R) system in Micromedex Inc, Englewood, Colorado (edition expired June 1999).

15 Vutyanavich T, Wongtrangan S and Ruangsri R (1995) Pyridoxine for nausea and vomiting of pregnancy: a randomised, double-blind, placebo-controlled study. *Am J Obstet Gynecol.* **173**: 881–4.

16 Sahakian V, Rouse D, Sipes SL *et al.* (1991) Vitamin B$_6$ is effective therapy for nausea and vomiting of pregnancy: a randomised, double-blind, placebo-controlled study. *Obstet Gynecol.* **78**: 33–6.

17 Guikontes E, Spantideas A and Kiakakis J (1992) Ondansetron and hyperemesis gravidarum. *Lancet.* **340**: 1223.

18 World MJ (1993) Ondansetron and hyperemesis gravidarum. *Lancet.* **341**: 185.

19 Sullivan CA, Johnson CA, Roach H *et al.* (1996) A pilot study of intravenous ondansetron for hyperemesis gravidarum. *Am J Obstet Gynecol.* **174**: 1565–8.

20 Nelson-Piercy C and de Swiet M (1994) Corticosteroids for the treatment of hyperemesis gravidarum. *Br J Obstet Gynaecol.* **101**: 1013–5.

21 Nelson-Piercy C and de Swiet M (1995) Complications of the use of corticosteroids for the treatment of hyperemesis gravidarum. *Br J Obstet Gynaecol.* **102**: 508–9.

22 Taylor R (1996) Successful management of hyperemesis gravidarum using steroid therapy. *Quart J Med.* **89**: 103–7.

23 Rubin PC, Craig GF, Gavin K *et al.* (1986) Prospective survey of use of therapeutic drugs, alcohol and cigarettes during pregnancy. *BMJ.* **292**: 81–3.

24 Corby DG (1978) Aspirin and pregnancy: maternal and fetal effects. *Pediatrics.* **62**(Suppl): 930–7.

25 CLASP Collaborative Group (1995) Low-dose aspirin in pregnancy and early childhood development: follow-up of the collaborative low-dose aspirin study in pregnancy. *Br J Obstet Gynaecol.* **102**: 861–8.

26 Prasad RNV (1982) Prostaglandin synthetase inhibitors and their effects on the fetus and the newborn. *Ann Acad Med.* **11**(4): 513–20.

27 van der Heijden BJ, Carlus C, Narcy F *et al.* (1994) Persistent anuria, neonatal death and renal microcystic lesions after prenatal exposure to indomethacin. *Am J Obstet Gynecol.* **171**: 617–23.

28 Torfs CP, Katz EA, Bateson TF *et al.* (1996) Maternal medications and environmental exposures as risk factors for gastroschisis. *Teratology.* **54**: 84–92.

29 Mangurten HH and Benawra R (1980) Neonatal codeine withdrawal in infants of non-addicted mothers. *Pediatrics.* **65**: 159–60.

30 Ruggins NR, Watkins S and Rutter N (1992) An unusual cause of convulsions in a newborn infant. *Eur J Pediatr.* **151**: 918.

31 Rathmell JP, Viscomi CM and Ashburn MA (1997) Management of non-obstetric pain during pregnancy and lactation. *Anesth Analges.* **85**: 1074–87.

32 Anon (1990) Heartburn in pregnancy. *Drug Ther Bull.* **28**: 11–12.

33 Enkin M, Keirse MJNC, Renfrew M *et al.* (1995) *A Guide to Effective Care in Pregnancy and Childbirth* (2nd edn). Oxford Univeristy Press, Oxford.

34 Jewell DJ and Young G (1999) Interventions for treating constipation in pregnancy (Cochrane review). In *The Cochrane Library,* Issue 1. Update Software, Oxford.

35 Lewis JH and Weingold AB (1985) The use of gastrointestinal drugs during pregnancy and lactation. *Am J Gastroenterol.* **80**: 912–23.

36 Sullivan C and Smith LG (1993) Management of vulvovaginitis in pregnancy. *Clin Obstet Gynaecol.* **36**: 195–205.

37 Rosa FW, Baum C and Shaw M (1987) Pregnancy outcomes after first-trimester vaginitis drug therapy. *Obstet Gynecol.* **69**: 751–5.

38 Piper JM, Mitchel EF and Ray WA (1993) Prenatal use of metronidazole and birth defects: no association. *Obstet Gynecol.* **82**: 348–52.

39 Burtin P, Taddio A, Ariburnu O *et al.* (1995) Safety of metronidazole in pregnancy: a meta-analysis. *Am J Obstet Gynecol.* **172**: 525–9.

40 Young G and Jewell DJ (1999) Interventions for leg cramps in pregnancy (Cochrane review). In *The Cochrane Library*, Issue 1. Update Software, Oxford.

41 Pfaffenrath V and Rehm M (1998) Migraine in pregnancy. What are the safest treatment options? *Drug Safety.* **19**(5): 383–8.

42 Shuhaiber S, Pastuszak A, Schick B *et al.* (1998) Pregnancy outcome following first-trimester exposure to sumatriptan. *Neurology.* **51**(2): 581–3.

43 Leach FN (1990) Management of threadworm infestation during pregnancy. *Arch Dis Child.* **65**(4): 399–400.

44 de Silva N, Guyatt H and Bundy D (1997) Anthelmintics. A comparative review of their clinical pharmacology. *Drugs.* **53**(5): 769–88.

45 de Silva NR, Sirisena JLGJ, Gunasekera DPS *et al.* (1999) Effect of mebendazole therapy during pregnancy on birth outcome. *Lancet.* **353**: 1145–9.

46 Malathion document in TERIS Hall AH (ed) in Reprorisk (R) system in Micromedex Inc, Englewood, Colorado (edition expired June 1999).

47 Permethrin document in TERIS Hall AH (ed) in Reprorisk (R) system in Micromedex Inc, Englewood, Colorado (edition expired June 1999).

CHAPTER FOUR

Common problems in the lactating woman

Sally Inch

Many women will experience some pain and/or discomfort in the days following childbirth. Although drug treatment is often unnecessary, there are some situations where symptom relief will benefit the mother without detrimental effects on the breastfeeding infant. Conditions for which treatment may be necessary include perineal pain, uterine pain (afterpains), constipation, nipple pain, uterine infection, breast pain (engorgement and mastitis) and nipple and/or breast infection.

Perineal and uterine pain

Paracetamol is the analgesic of choice in breastfeeding. The amounts that pass into breast milk are considered too small to be harmful.[1] If necessary it may be given in combination with codeine (as co-codamol) or dextropropoxyphene (co-proxamol), both of which are considered compatible with breastfeeding.[2] With codeine there is the possibility of constipation in the mother and a small risk of colic or constipation in the baby.[2]

Non-steroidal anti-inflammatory drugs (NSAIDs), such as ibuprofen and diclofenac, may be used for more severe pain and for conditions associated with inflammation, such as mastitis. All these compounds appear in breast milk in concentrations too small to be harmful to the infant.[3] Aspirin is not recommended in breastfeeding. In general the risk to the infant is low, although high doses may disturb platelet function. However, children under the age of 12 should not be exposed to aspirin because of the increased risk of Reye's syndrome.[3,4]

Topical applications may be useful for perineal pain. The use of lignocaine has been assessed in the context of clinical trials. The analgesic effect of 5% aqueous lignocaine (lidocaine) was equivalent to a single 500 mg dose of mefenamic acid. Lignocaine (lidocaine) should not be given in combination with topical steroids as it may delay healing.[5]

Constipation

It is common for bowel activity to be reduced in the first few days following delivery. Unless the mother is uncomfortable, reassurance may be all that is necessary, together with appropriate dietary advice such as increasing the intake of fibre-rich foods and fluids.

If treatment is necessary, the agents that are preferred for use during pregnancy, such as the bulking agents ispaghula husk or sterculia, are first choice. The mother should be advised that the full effect may take some days to develop. Osmotic laxatives, such as lactulose, are also suitable although they also take up to 48 hours to work. Glycerin suppositories have a local action and therefore pose no problem for the breastfed infant. Stimulant laxatives, such as senna and bisacodyl, may cause colic and/or diarrhoea in the infant and should be avoided. Faecal softeners, such as liquid paraffin, should also be avoided.

Nipple pain

In the early days this is nearly always due to poor attachment of the baby at the breast. If the baby is not enabled to take a big enough mouthful of breast tissue, the mother's nipple will be compressed between the baby's tongue and hard palate. No cream, spray or gel will heal a nipple that is being repeatedly damaged by poor attachment and none have been shown in the context of controlled trials to have any beneficial effect.[6] The 'treatment' is to teach the mother how to apply the principles of good attachment.

Nipple damage

Poor attachment can often give rise to damage as well as pain. If the skin is broken to the point where it forms a scab and/or sticks to clothing between feeds, the use of paraffin-impregnated gauze (Jelonet, Intertulle) may be used to prevent the surface epithelium from drying out and thus provides the appropriate environment for 'moist wound healing'.[7] This will reduce the trauma to the nipple as it is stretched (along with the breast tissue) to form in the infant's mouth; but only removing the cause of the damage (i.e. improving attachment) will permit the nipple to heal. Damage which does not heal in spite of improved attachment may be due to secondary infection, either bacterial or fungal. Topical treatment is often sufficient; sodium fusidate 2% (Fucidin) as a cream or a gauze dressing (Fucidin intertulle) may be applied to the nipple after feeds for five to seven days. For topical thrush treatment, *see* below.

Nipple thrush

Nipple pain that suddenly appears after a period of pain-free feeding is often due to thrush. This condition is becoming more common and often follows antibiotic use.[8] Characteristically, the mother complains of a burning sensation, intense itching or severe nipple pain that increases as a breastfeed continues or appears after the feed. (This is in contrast to the pain from poor attachment which is usually present from the start of the feed.) The sensations may be present for some time after the feed and the mother may find even the touch of clothing distressing. Both nipples are likely to be affected. The appearance of the nipples may be unchanged from their normal state, although there may be a pale area around the base of the nipple/areola, which may be slightly oedematous. The baby may or may not have obvious oral thrush, characterised by white patches on the sides of the mouth, inside the lips or at the back of the tongue. The baby may pull off the breast while feeding and seem fretful or uncomfortable if his/her mouth is sore. The baby may also have perianal thrush.

In the absence of any visible sign in either mother or baby, diagnosis is made on the basis of the symptoms having excluded poor attachment as the cause of the pain. However, poor attachment and nipple thrush may coexist. Both the mother and the baby will need to be treated concurrently, or reinfection will occur. Miconazole 2% cream should be applied to the nipples after every breastfeed and (as an oral gel) to the baby's mouth four times a day after feeds. Treatment should be continued for at least two weeks, although the pain should disappear within two to three days. Nystatin, which may be used similarly, seems to be less effective.

Gentian (crystal) violet is an antiseptic dye which has some efficacy in the management of candida infections. It is still widely used in the USA as an oral paediatric aqueous solution (0.25–0.5%) used once a day for no more than three days. However, ingestion of gentian violet can cause nausea, vomiting, diarrhoea and abdominal pain. Topical application of high concentrations can cause ulceration and skin necrosis. In addition, animal studies give rise to concerns about carcinogenicity. For these reasons the use of topical gentian violet cannot be advocated.

Thrush in the breast

Most deep breast pain is caused by inefficient milk removal secondary to poor attachment, and not by ductal thrush. Evidence of nipple thrush would be expected prior to breast infiltration, although this is not always the case. Mothers often describe the pain in the breast as 'shooting pain' which goes through to the back and shoulder. This pain is usually worse toward the end of the feeding and worsens still after the feeding is over. It also tends to be much worse at night. If intense deep breast pain between feeds persists in spite of good attachment and topical treatment, systemic treatment will be required.

Oral treatment consists of either nystatin (500 000 units every six hours for 14 days) or fluconazole (150 mg initially followed by 50 mg twice a day for 10 days). Neither is licensed for this use in the UK, although both may be used in neonates. Nystatin is poorly absorbed and consequently very little will appear in the mother's milk. In contrast, 90% of an oral dose of fluconazole is absorbed and clinical cure rates in oral candidiasis are significantly higher than those achieved with nystatin. Fluconazole appears in breast milk at similar concentrations to those in plasma. Published data on its effects on the nursing infant are extremely limited. However, no reports of problems have been found and it appears to be widely used in the USA with no suggestion of adverse effects in the infant.[9] Oral fluconazole may be appropriate treatment for some women with symptoms strongly suggestive of breast thrush, although the lack of published safety and efficacy data should be borne in mind.

Uterine infection

Post-partum infection may be suspected if the lochia is persistently red or smells offensive, if the mother complains of suprapubic pain or feels generally unwell, or if the uterus is slow to involute. As with other systemic infections (*see* Chapter 11), treatment should be with an appropriately sensitive antibiotic. Whilst waiting for high vaginal swab (HVS) culture, a broad-spectrum penicillin, cephalosporin or co-amoxiclav should be given.

Engorgement

Breast engorgement is common in the first few days after birth; women experience a sense of fullness, warmth and heaviness of the breasts as the vascular supply to the breasts increases. If milk is not removed as it is formed, the alveolar space (into which the cells secrete milk) can become overdistended, accompanied by tender, swollen and painful breasts. This problem was more likely when restrictions were placed on the duration and frequency of feeds. These days its appearance should alert the health professional(s) caring for the mother to pay greater attention to the way in which the mother is attaching her baby to her breast, since it is almost certainly caused by inefficient breast use. All of both breasts are firm, oedematous, painful (somctimes flushed) and may have an orange peel appearance. However, recent data indicate that painful breasts and nipples remain an important contributing factor in women giving up breastfeeding in the first few weeks post-delivery.[10] There are many non-drug treatments for engorgement ranging from massage, application of heat, ice packs and medicinal plant remedies such as cabbage leaves. In some cultures the application of cool cabbage leaves to the breast has been a remedy for engorgement for many years. The mechanism of efficacy is uncertain. One small study suggests that using cabbage leaves may result in fewer women stopping breastfeeding, although further research is needed to confirm this.[11] The large outer leaves of a leafy cabbage should be cooled in a refrigerator or freezer before applying them to the breasts for a short period of time. This practice may bring some relief to the mother in the early days of breastfeeding and there is no reason to suppose that it is harmful. An anti-inflammatory analgesic (*see* above) may also be required while the cause of the problem is treated.

Mastitis

A lactating woman with a swollen, red and painful area on her breast, sometimes with a raised pulse and temperature and even a flu-like feeling often accompanied by shivering attacks/rigors, is readily diagnosed as suffering from mastitis. In the majority of cases no infection is present and the symptoms are those of unrelieved milk stasis.[12–15]

Typically, it occurs in the early weeks when the mother is learning the skills of good attachment and on the side opposite the mother's preferred side for holding her baby, as most mothers are less able to put the baby to the breast efficiently with the hand that usually holds the baby, compared with the hand that is usually free to perform tasks.[16]

Inflammation and infection, although separate entities, often coexist and the common extension of the suffix 'itis' (which actually means inflammation) to mean infection (as in appendicitis, bronchitis, peritonitis) has tended to result in 'mastitis' being thought of inevitably as a breast infection. This view is regularly reinforced by the observation that the mastitis improves when antibiotics are given. In the absence of infection this improvement may be due to an anti-inflammatory action that antibiotics can exert.[17] The lactating breast is protected from infection in several ways:

- the removal of the milk from the breasts as it is formed denies bacteria the conditions needed to multiply significantly
- the natural direction of flow of the milk along the ducts tends to wash organisms out of the breast

- antimicrobial factors present in the breast milk help to protect the breast against infection, particularly with *Staphylococcus aureus*.

However, if the free drainage of milk from a section of breast is obstructed, the milk collects in the alveoli and the pressure begins to rise. The distension in the alveoli can often be felt as a lump in the breast tissue and is tender when palpated. If this distension is not relieved, the pressure in the alveoli may rise to the point where substances from the milk are forced through the cell walls and into connective tissue. This will cause diffuse heat and redness over an area of the breast. If the milk also makes its way via breast capillaries into the bloodstream, then the mother's temperature may begin to rise and she may develop flu-like symptoms and even rigors, similar to those observed in patients having an incompatible blood transfusion, i.e. an immune response to a foreign substance.[18]

In most instances mastitis is the result of inefficient or ineffective milk removal. If this is remedied quickly, the mastitis should resolve without further treatment. A delay in addressing the cause of the problem may result in superimposed infection, particularly if the skin is damaged. This is made more likely if the raised alveolar pressure is exacerbated by the abrupt cessation of breastfeeding.[12,14,19,20]

Although demonstrated that a differential diagnosis between infectious and non-infectious mastitis can be made on the basis of a leucocyte and bacterial count, this facility is rarely available.[14] A rule of thumb, in the absence of rapid differential diagnosis, is to address the underlying cause and improve milk removal and to begin antibiotics if there is no improvement within 8 to 24 hours.[16,21–23] However, if it is accepted that inefficient breast 'drainage' rather than infection, is the underlying reason for the mastitis, observation and correction of the mother's feeding technique must become an integral part of the management of this distressing and painful condition. The mother may be destined to make repeated trips to the surgery if only her symptoms are treated.

Choice of antibiotic

The most commonly isolated organism in confirmed cases of breast infection or abscess formation is *Staphylococcus aureus*. In the absence of a milk culture to guide prescription it would be reasonable to assume that this is the offending organism. Many strains of *Staphylococcus pyogenes* are now resistant to penicillin, particularly those that are acquired in hospital. It would thus be advisable to use an antibiotic (or a combination of antibiotics) to which *S. aureus* is likely to be sensitive but which is not in common use in hospitals. Cefalexin seems to be the most widely recommended antibiotic.[23–25] It is better tolerated than erythromycin and causes fewer gastrointestinal disturbances in the mother and infant.[25,26] It is secreted into breast milk in low concentrations, with milk levels averaging 0.5 mL (therapeutic range in serum, 2–64 g/mL), and is considered safe for use if breastfeeding.[27,28]

Flucloxacillin is also widely used and is safe.[23,25,29] Erythromycin may also be effective but is more likely to cause gastrointestinal upset in mother and/or baby.[23,25,29] It is also less favoured because of increasing numbers of erythromycin-resistant strains of *S. aureus* (28%).[26] Although no specific problems have been reported, with any antibiotic the effects on the infant bowel flora and the possibility of allergy must be kept in mind.

Breast abscess

Good management of mastitis should prevent progression to abscess formation, but if breast abscess is suspected a firm diagnosis can be made with the use of ultrasound or aspiration.[29,30] Confirmation should be followed by aspiration or incision and drainage. Antibiotics should be given (guided by culture studies if possible) and breastfeeding should continue.

Antibiotics alone are unlikely to be of value[31] considering that, as in any suppurative process, the lactating breast responds by localising the infection by forming an antibiotic-impermeable granulation tissue barrier (possibly the result of the interaction of coagulase [produced by the bacteria] and plasma fibrinogen, resulting in fibrin, which is deposited in the tissues), thus protecting the pathogenic bacteria from the body's defence system.[32] This effectively results in impairment of vascular perfusion and poor antibiotic levels at the abscess site and has been the rationale for the treatment of breast abscess by incision, curettage and primary suture.[32–34] This involves the evacuation of pus, the destruction of the granulation tissue and the obliteration of the abscess cavity by deep mattress sutures.[32]

In 1988, Dixon reported on the outcome of six lactating women with large abscesses (15–40 mL pus) in whom the treatment was continued breastfeeding and aspiration of the abscess with a large-bore 919-gauge needle every day until it resolved.[33] This is now a widely used procedure as it is much less painful and mutilating than incision and drainage.[35] No formal comparison has yet been made between open drainage and aspiration. There is an impression that aspiration may not drain the pus that continues to form fast enough to prevent spontaneous rupture (Woolridge, personal communication). Against this has to be set the advantages of a procedure done on an out-patient basis under local anaesthesia and which causes minimal breast disfiguration. In the absence of a better basis for treatment selection, the mother should be offered the choice.

The importance of continued breast drainage/breastfeeding

The impression gained from uncontrolled studies was that if mastitis (or even abscess) does occur, the outcome is better if lactation (and breast drainage) continue.[12,19,20,36-39] This was confirmed in the context of the only randomised controlled trial to date in which mothers who were suffering from both infectious and non-infectious mastitis, and who expressed their breast after a feed, fared better than those who did not.[14]

Outcome for the infant feeding from the affected breast

In most cases of mastitis there is no demonstrable infectious process, but even when *S. aureus* is present in the milk it appears to do the infant no harm, even if the mother develops an abscess.[12,15,19,40-43] However, some mothers may prefer to express and discard the milk from the affected breast while healing takes place and others will be unable to breastfeed because of the site of the abscess.

Other postnatal considerations in relation to breastfeeding

Anaesthesia in the postnatal period

The most commonly used anaesthetic agents are gases, such as nitrous oxide, and volatile liquid anaesthetics. Nitrous oxide is eliminated within three to five minutes of ceasing to breathe the gas; no data exist on its passage into breast milk, but it would seem unlikely.[2] Halogenated anaesthetic agents (halothane, enflurane, methoxyflurane and isoflurane) are frequently used as supplements to nitrous oxide. A large proportion of halothane (60–80%) is rapidly excreted by exhalation and only 15% is metabolised by the liver.[2] The amount to which the infant would be exposed may be regarded as negligible. All of these anaesthetic agents have been assessed in relation to their effect on neonates whose mothers underwent elective caesarean section and no ill-effects have been reported.[44] These agents are compatible with breastfeeding. Thiopentone sodium, a short-acting barbiturate that is often used as an induction agent, has been studied in relation to post-operative levels in breast milk and colostrum.[3] The maximum recorded levels were considered insignificant. Other drugs, such as narcotic analgesics and benzodiazepines, may be used in conjunction with anaesthetics and their use is considered elsewhere.

Local anaesthetics

Lignocaine's (lidocaine) use in breastfeeding is approved by the American Academy of Pediatrics. Small doses of local anaesthetics are used for dental and other minor surgical procedures; the amount passing into breastmilk is insignificant and absorption after oral administration is very poor anyway.[2] Furthermore, these agents are usually given with adrenaline (epinephrine) which limits their entry into the bloodstream.[45] If given via the caudal or epidual route, amounts up to 300 mg are considered compatible with breastfeeding.[46]

Hormonal methods of contraception

Where possible, breastfeeding mothers should be encouraged to use non-hormonal methods of contraception. The long-term effects of exposing infants, particularly male infants, to female hormones is not known, but the amounts passing into breast milk are small. Oestrogens have the potential to suppress lactation so progestogen-only oral contraceptives are preferred.[3] This may decrease the mother's milk supply briefly, so she may need to offer the breast more frequently for a few days. The progestogen-only pill may be taken from three weeks after the birth.

References

1 Bitzen PO, Gustafsson B, Jostell KG et al. (1981) Excretion of paracetamol in human breast milk. Eur J Clin Pharm. **20**: 123–5.

2 Hale T (1998) Medications and Mothers' Milk (6th edn). Pharmasoft Medical Publishing, Texas.

3 Anderson PO (1991) Therapy review: drug use during breastfeeding. Clin Pharm. **10**: 594–624.

4 Bennet PN (1996) Drugs and Human Lactation (2nd edn). Elsevier, Amsterdam.

5 Sleep J (1990) Postnatal perineal care. In Postnatal Care: a research-based approach (eds V Levy, J Alexander and S Roch). MacMillan, London.

6 Inch S and Renfrew MJ (1989) Common breastfeeding problems. In Effective Care in Pregnancy and Childbirth (eds M Enkin, I Chalmers and M Kierse). Oxford University Press, Oxford.

7 Cable B, Stewart M and Davis J (1997) Nipple wound care: a new approach to an old problem. J Hum Lact. **13**(4): 313–18.

8 Amir L (1991) Patient education. Mastitis. Aust Fam Physic. **20**(6): 841.

9 Newman J (1998) Handout No. 20. Fluconazole. Written by Jack Newman, MD FRCPC (http://www.thenaturalway.org). (May be copied and distributed without further permission.)

10 Foster K, Lader D and Cheesbrough S (1997) Infant Feeding 1995: survey carried out by the Office for National Statistics, p. 25. The Stationery Office, London.

11 Renfrew M and Lang S (1999) Cabbage leaves for breast engorgement (Cochrane review). *The Cochrane Library*, Issue 1. Update Software, Oxford.

12 Marshall BR, Hepper JK and Zirbel CC (1975) Sporadic puerperal mastitis: an infection that need not interrupt lactation. *J Am Med Assoc.* **233**: 1377–9.

13 Neibyl J, Spence MR and Parmley TH (1978) Sporadic (non-epidemic) puerperal mastitis. *J Reprod Med.* **20**(2): 97–100.

14 Thomsen AC, Espersen T and Maigaard S (1984) Course and treatment of milk stasis, non-infectious inflammation of the breast and infectious mastitis in nursing women. *Am J Obstet Gynecol.* **149**(5): 492–5.

15 Matheson I, Aursnes I, Horgen M *et al.* (1988) Bacterilogical findings and clinical symptoms in relation to clinical outcome in puerperal mastitis. *Acta Obstet Gynecol Scand.* **67**: 723–6.

16 Inch S and Fisher C (1994) Mastitis in lactating women. *Practitioner.* **239**: 472–6.

17 Spector WG and Willoughby DA (1974) *Inflammation: useful and non-useful. Folia traumatologica*, p. 15. Ciba-Giegy Ltd, Switzerland.

18 Gunther M (1958) Discussion on the breast in pregnancy and lactation. *Proc Roy Soc Med.* **51**: 306–9.

19 Kimball ER (1951) Breastfeeding in private practice. *Northwestern Univ Med Sch Bull.* **25**: 257.

20 Newton M (1950) Breast abscess as a result of lactation failure. *Surg Gynecol Obstet.* **91**: 651–5.

21 Minchin M (1989) *Breastfeeding Matters*, pp. 150–65. Alma Publications and George Unwin, Australia.

22 Royal College of Midwives (1991) *Successful Breastfeeding* (2nd edn). Churchill Livingstone, Edinburgh.

23 Amir L (1993) *Mastitis* [handout] *Aust Lact Consult Assoc News.* **4**(3): 117.

24 Riordan J (1983) *A Practical Guide to Breastfeeding*, pp. 149–56. CV Mosby, St Louis.

25 Cigolini MC (1995) *Mastitis: the big picture*. Seminar paper presented at: Breastfeeding – getting it right. Held at Sydney Marriott Hotel, Sydney, Australia, March 30, 1995. Seminar organised and papers published by Nursing Mothers' Association of Australia.

26 Turnbridge J (1995) What to use instead of flucloxacillin [editorial]. *Aust Prescrib.* **18**(3): 54–5.

27 Ogle KS and Davis S (1988) Mastitis in lactating women [clinical conference]. *J Fam Pract.* **26**(2): 139–44.

28 Fulton B and Moore LL (1992) Anti-infectives in breast milk. Part 1. Penicillins and cephalosporins. *J Hum Lact.* **8**(3): 157–8.

29 Dixon JM (1994) ABC of breast diseases: breast infection. *BMJ.* **309**: 946–8.

30 Hayes R, Michell M and Nunnerley HB (1991) Acute inflammation of the breast: the role of breast ultrasound in diagnosis and mangement. *Clin Radiol.* **44**(4): 2536.

31 Rench MA and Baker CJ (1989) Group B streptococcal breast in a mother and mastitis in her infant. *Obstet Gynecol.* **73**(5, Pt 2): 875–7.

32 Benson EA and Goodman MA (1970) Incision with primary suture in the treatment of acute puerperal breast abscess. *Br J Surg.* **57**(1): 55–8.

33 Dixon JM (1988) Repeated aspiration of breast abscesses in lactating women. *BMJ.* **297**: 1517–18.

34 Qureshi F (1982) The acute breast abscess: practical procedures. *Aust Fam Physic.* **11**(3): 2134.

35 Lawlor Smith C (1994) Treating mastitis [letter comment]. *Aust Fam Physic.* **23**(1): 77; **23**(5): 9789; **23**(7): 1388.

36 Benson EA and Goodman MA (1970) An evaluation of the use of stilboestrol and antibiotics in the early management of acute puerpural breast abscess. *Br J Surg.* **57**(1): 225–58.

37 Newton M and Newton N (1962) The normal course and managment of labour. *Clin Obstet Gynecol.* **5**(1): 44–63.

38 Riordan J and Auerbach KG (1993) *Breastfeeding and Human Lactation.* Jones & Bartlett, Boston, Massachusetts.

39 Walsh A (1949) Acute mastitis. *Lancet.* **2**: 635–9.

40 Duncan JT and Walker J (1942) *Staphlococcus aureus* in the milk of nursing mothers and the alimentary canal of their infants: a report to the Medical Research Council. *J Hyg.* **42**: 474.

41 Taylor MD and Way S (1946) Penicillin treatment of acute puerperal mastitis. *BMJ.* **Nov 16**, 731–2.

42 Jeffrey JS (1947) Treatment of acute puerpural mastitis. *Edinb Med J.* **54**: 442–6.

43 Devereux WP (1970) Acute puerperal mastitis: evaluation of its management. *Am J Obstet Gynaecol.* **108**(1): 7881.

44 Warren TM, Dattas S, Ostheimer GW *et al.* (1983) Comparison of the maternal and neonatal effects of halothane, enflurane and isoflurane for caesarean delivery. *Anesth Analges.* **62**: 516–20.

45 Benz J (1997) Anesthetic use during breastfeeding. *J Hum Lact.* **13**(4): 313–18.

46 Zeisler JA, Gaarder TD and De Mesquita SA (1986) Lidocaine excretion in breast milk. *Drug Intell Clin Pharm.* **20**: 691–3.

CHAPTER FIVE

Gastrointestinal disorders

Rodney Taylor

Treatment of specific diseases in pregnancy

Gastrointestinal complaints are common during pregnancy. The majority are usually self-limiting and respond to reassurance, dietary change and simple remedies. Common complaints are heartburn and dyspepsia, abdominal discomfort and constipation. The management of these is discussed in Chapter 3 'Common problems in pregnancy'. This chapter covers those conditions which are less commonly encountered during pregnancy (*see* list below).

The management of digestive diseases in pregnancy presents additional challenges and requires close collaboration between the obstetrician, gastroenterologist and general practitioner (GP), as well as all others involved. The course of pre-existing disease may be modified by pregnancy and require changes in treatment. A more difficult situation is when new digestive disease presents in pregnancy because its features may easily be dismissed, misdiagnosed or attributed to the effects of pregnancy.

The following conditions may pre-exist or present in pregnancy and require active treatment:

- oesophagitis, gastritis and duodenitis
- peptic ulceration +/– *Helicobacter pylori*
- gluten-sensitive enteropathy (coeliac disease)
- hepatobiliary disease
- hepatitis
- cholelithiasis
- cholestasis
- pancreatic disease

- acute pancreatitis
- chronic pancreatitis
- inflammatory bowel disease
- ulcerative colitis
- Crohn's disease
- gastrointestinal infections and infestations
- irritable bowel syndrome
- gastrointestinal malignancy
- haemorrhoids.

Oesophagitis, gastritis and duodenitis

These inflammatory changes in the upper gastrointestinal tract usually present with dyspeptic symptoms such as heartburn, waterbrash, dysphagia, epigastric discomfort, flatulence, bloating and distension, which are often meal related. Dyspeptic symptoms are common in pregnancy, occurring in up to 80% of women. They usually respond to dietary changes and simple antacids (*see* Chapter 3). If symptoms are severe or resistant to treatment then further investigation may be necessary. Upper gastrointestinal endoscopy is the investigation of choice. The confirmatory diagnosis is usually made at endoscopy, which is safe in pregnancy in experienced hands. Barium studies are contraindicated in pregnancy due to the radiation risk. The management of these symptoms is discussed in Chapter 3.

Peptic ulceration +/– *Helicobacter pylori*

Peptic ulceration is uncommon in pregnancy; the diagnosis can only be confirmed by endoscopy.[1] The symptoms are similar to those of non-ulcer dyspepsia. Ulcers will heal well with antacids in adequate high dosage for sufficient time and this is the safest treatment in pregnancy. Safety data on H_2-receptor antagonists and proton pump inhibitors is limited, so their use in pregnancy is discouraged.[2–4] If *Helicobacter pylori* is present (as shown by serology, biopsy or CLO-test, but not by radioactive breath test), treatment is best deferred until after delivery. There is no evidence that the main groups of drugs used for *H. pylori* eradication (i.e. metronidazole, penicillins, H_2-receptor antagonists and proton pump inhibitors) have harmful effects on the fetus, however, so women who have been exposed inadvertently may be reassured.

Gluten-sensitive enteropathy (GSE) or coeliac disease

This may present for the first time in pregnancy, as diarrhoea, often with weight loss and evidence of malabsorption, but is more likely to pre-exist.[1] If it is not adequately treated it results in maternal anaemia and a malnourished fetus. The diagnosis is confirmed by the appearance of partial or total villous atrophy seen on jejunal or low duodenal biopsy. Adherence to a gluten-free diet results in recovery of the villous pattern and resolution of symptoms. The increased nutritional demands of pregnancy can create difficulties and involvement of a dietician is advisable. This diet must be continued throughout pregnancy and any nutritional deficiencies can be corrected safely with dietary supplements.

Hepatobiliary disease

There are many complex physiological changes in hepatic and biliary function associated with pregnancy which make the diagnosis of hepatobiliary disease difficult.[5] Some diseases of the liver and biliary tree are peculiar to pregnancy and others are coincidental. Many are serious and potentially life threatening for the mother and the fetus. Early, safe diagnosis is essential to ensure that appropriate treatment is initiated as soon as possible. The management of these diseases, and related prescribing, is specialised and must be dealt with in collaboration with tertiary referral centres.

This especially applies to acute fatty liver of pregnancy, liver disease associated with hypertension or hyperemesis, and HELLP (haemolysis, elevated liver enzymes and low platelet count) syndrome; all need referral to a specialist unit.

Hepatitis is the commonest cause of jaundice in pregnancy and is usually viral, most commonly hepatitis A or B:

A – from contaminated water or food
B – drug abuse, sexual transmission or blood transfusion abroad
C – blood transfusion
D – sexually transmitted with B
E – epidemic in some tropical areas.

It always requires specialist management. In general, treatment is as in the non-pregnant woman, but interferon is contraindicated in pregnancy because of limited experience and concerns about its immunological effect on the fetus.

The treatments of acute liver failure, cirrhosis, chronic active hepatitis, primary biliary cirrhosis and Wilson's disease are also the same as those in the non-pregnant patient, accepting the potential risks.[2,6] Oesophageal varices may be safely sclerosed as a risk-reducing measure. Liver transplantation, and the required immunosuppression, is a specialist tertiary referral issue.

Cholelithiasis

If gallstones precipitate cholecystitis in pregnancy, surgery can be used if necessary, although medical management is preferable, using IV fluids and either an oral cephalosporin or IV gentamicin. If gentamicin is used, serum levels must be carefully monitored as there is a risk of toxicity to both mother and fetus. Bile acid dissolution is not considered safe.[5]

Cholestasis

Intrahepatic cholestasis of pregnancy is the second most common cause of jaundice in pregnancy after viral hepatitis. It carries a high risk of fetal distress and a significant chance of stillbirth. It usually presents with mild jaundice, generalised pruritus, fatigue and sometimes abdominal discomfort.[5] If suspected, women should be referred urgently to an obstetrician. Patients should be screened to exclude autoimmune or viral hepatitis. Pruritus can be troublesome and may be helped by cholestyramine, which is considered to be safe.[7] Vitamin K injections reduce the risk of haemorrhage associated with disordered blood clotting.

Pancreatic disease

There are changes in the pancreas in pregnancy which make interpretation of serum amylase, lipase and triglyceride levels difficult, but pancreatic disease is relatively rare. Acute pancreatitis is an uncommon cause of abdominal pain in pregnancy, but if it occurs it can be severe and life threatening. Management is as in the non-pregnant patient, aiming to rest the pancreas and gut, provide nutritional support and minimise complications.[5,8] There are few drugs used in treatment; their benefits are equivocal and their safety in pregnancy is unknown. The key is meticulous attention to fluid and electrolyte balances, trace elements and supportive measures. Total parenteral nutrition can be used safely in pregnancy.

Chronic pancreatitis is characterised by exocrine insufficiency and often some endocrine deficiency resulting in diabetes. Pancreatic enzyme supplements allow normal digestion and absorption, and are safe in pregnancy. Diabetic control should be meticulous and maintained with insulin during pregnancy. Oral hypoglycaemic agents should be discontinued preconceptually or as soon as pregnancy is recognised (*see* Chapter 12). Dietetic support is essential to ensure good nutrition and diabetic control.

Cystic fibrosis is now treated much more effectively and many patients live into healthy adulthood. Their treatment to prevent respiratory problems, supplement pancreatic exocrine insufficiency and possibly control diabetes with insulin must be maintained in pregnancy in consultation with their physician. Good control of fluid and electrolytes is essential. The breast milk of women with cystic fibrosis has a high sodium content but that is not a contraindication to breastfeeding.[9]

Inflammatory bowel disease (IBD)

IBD may develop in pregnancy but is more likely to be pre-existing, and probably already diagnosed and treated. Fertility is normal if disease control is good. Patients who plan conception should be encouraged to do so when in stable remission.[10–12] The major forms of IBD are ulcerative colitis, in which inflammation is confined to the colonic mucosa; Crohn's disease, which can affect any part of the bowel but has a predilection for the terminal ileum and can cause strictures and fistulae; and non-specific colitis and proctitis. All patients may require surgery at some stage but most of their management is medical and is similar for the different conditions.

There is a complex interplay between the disease and pregnancy. Ulcerative colitis may present in the first trimester, which limits the use of investigative techniques, particularly radiology, and makes diagnosis difficult. Many patients improve in the second and third trimester, particularly those with ulcerative colitis, but are prone to relapse after delivery.[10–13] Crohn's disease generally has a more erratic and unpredictable course, especially in pregnancy.[14] Generally, pregnancy has no deleterious effect on IBD and if the disease is well controlled it has limited effect on pregnancy. Birth weights may be reduced in Crohn's disease. Treatment of IBD aims to control inflammation by using three major therapeutic agents: corticosteroids (oral prednisolone, oral budesonide, or IV hydrocortisone in an exacerbation), 5-ASA derivatives (sulphasalazine, mesalazine, olsalazine) and azathioprine. There is considerable anecdotal experience now in the use of these drugs in pregnancy but limited published data. All appear to be safe in pregnancy.[15–18] The highest priority, both preconceptually and in pregnancy, is to obtain optimal and stable control with the lowest dosage regimen. The choice of treatment regimen is governed by what is most effective for the individual patient. Inflammatory markers and haematology need to be monitored regularly. Dosage should always be reduced to the lowest level that maintains remission and good health in the mother.

Gastrointestinal infections and infestations

Most gastrointestinal infections result in some form of gastroenteritis, with alteration of bowel habit (usually towards diarrhoea), abdominal discomfort, cramps or pain, nausea and/or vomiting. They are usually self-limiting and best treated with supportive measures. If symptoms are prolonged for more than 24–48 hours, stools should be examined for ova, cysts and parasites and microbial culture. Many episodes are due to enterotoxins or viruses, neither of which respond to antibiotics, which are best avoided even for proven bacterial infections. There is no indication for the routine use of antibiotics for gastrointestinal infections in pregnancy. By the time culture results are available the illness is often over, but it is important to monitor such infections for public health reasons.

Travellers' diarrhoea is acute in onset, usually during or shortly after foreign travel, and is frequently accompanied by nausea, bloating, cramps and fever. It can be caused by a multitude of bacteria and viruses which can contaminate food or water, but enterotoxogenic *Escherichia coli* is the commonest (up to 70%), followed by *Shigella* (up to 20%). Most cases are self-limiting and do not require medication. Antibiotic prophylaxis with doxycycline, trimethoprim or active treatment with ciprofloxacin is effective in reducing the incidence of travellers' diarrhoea, but all are contraindicated in pregnancy.

Campylobacter species can cause a particularly unpleasant acute diarrhoeal illness and can present a particular cross-infection risk to the fetus and the newborn child. Infection is usually from unpasteurised milk or inadequately cooked poultry, which should be avoided. Supportive measures, and strict hygiene to prevent spread, are essential. In severe cases, oral erythromycin for four weeks can be used safely. Chloramphenicol and gentamicin may occasionally be used in suspected systemic infection and pregnancy would not necessarily preclude their use. Antibiotics carry the added risk of precipitating antibiotic-associated colitis. If this does occur it must be treated with vancomycin, which can be used safely as long as serum levels are monitored to minimise the risk of damage to the fetus.[19] Listeriosis has given considerable cause for concern recently, because of the risk to the fetus (*see* Chapter 11). High-risk sources include pâté and soft cheeses. The febrile flu-like illness is treated safely in pregnancy with IV amoxycillin, ampicillin or erythromycin.

Gastrointestinal infections in the immunocompromised and those with HIV and AIDS need specialist support and advice on treatment from a dedicated centre.

Gastrointestinal infestations can be a cause of poor nutritional status in the mother, resulting in anaemia and other manifestations of malnutrition. They are difficult to treat in pregnancy and during breastfeeding because most of the drugs used are toxic. Drug treatment can almost invariably be delayed until after delivery in most cases, but malnutrition must be corrected with vitamin and haematinic supplements as required. The commonest infestations are giardia, hookworm, whipworm, roundworm, threadworm and tapeworm; which are particularly likely in those arriving from developing countries. The exceptions to these rules are treatment of giardiasis and of *Entamoeba histolytica* with metronidazole, which is safe, though other, commonly used agents have not been fully evaluated for use in pregnancy.

Irritable bowel syndrome

Constipation, diarrhoea or fluctuating bowel habit, often associated with abdominal discomfort or pain, are the features of irritable bowel syndrome. This may predate or develop in the pregnancy. Diagnosis is by exclusion of other causes of altered bowel habit. If it is new this may present diagnostic problems because of constraints on investigation in pregnancy.

Treatment aims to relieve the major symptoms. Avoidance of 'trigger' foods and simple dietary change may help. Bulking agents, with an adequate fluid intake, relieve constipation and are better tolerated than bran. Anticholinergic agents (dicyclomine and hyoscine) and smooth muscle relaxants (mebeverine and alverine) are not recommended in pregnancy because there is inadequate safety data.[7,20] Peppermint is widely used in confectionery and peppermint oil is probably safe, though pharmacological safety data is lacking.

Gastrointestinal malignancy

Malignant disease of the gastrointestinal tract is rare in women of child-bearing age, but there are cases recorded. Most likely sites are colorectal, pancreatic and gastric cancers, and intestinal lymphoma. Management is as in the non-pregnant woman in close consultation with the oncologist and surgeon. The prognosis is unchanged by pregnancy but the practical management may be more difficult. Chemotherapy is contraindicated until delivery or termination, and the baby should not be breastfed during chemotherapy.

Gastrointestinal drugs to avoid or use with caution in pregnancy

There are numerous drugs available for the treatment of gastrointestinal disease (Table 5.1). Many are widely used over-the-counter (OTC) preparations for controlling common symptoms. The general principle of cautious use in pregnancy applies to all of these and highlights the need for a comprehensive drug history, particularly in the crucial first trimester, including OTC drugs and those taken before pregnancy was recognised or confirmed.

Table 5.1:   Safety of drugs prescribed for the treatment of gastrointestinal disease in pregnancy

Drugs	Safety in pregnancy
5-ASA derivatives (sulphasalazine, mesalazine, olsalazine)	Appear safe
Anticholinergics (dicyclomine, hyoscine)	Inadequate evidence of safety – avoid
Azathioprine	Available data do not suggest increased risk. Risk–benefit may be acceptable in some cases
Mebendazole (albendazole)	Avoid in first trimester
Bile salts (cheno- and urso-deoxycholic acids)	Avoid
Cisapride	Inadequate evidence of safety – avoid
Corticosteroids	May be used – minimise dose
Domperidone	Inadequate evidence of safety – avoid
Histamine H_2-receptor antagonists	Available data do not suggest increased fetal risk – avoid in first trimester
Proton pump inhibitors (omeprazole, lanzoprazole, pantoprazole)	Inadequate evidence of safety – avoid
Metoclopramide	May be used with caution
Metronidazole	Avoid high-dose regimens
Misoprostol	Contraindicated. Increases uterine tone, precipitates labour
Octreotide	Lack of data – avoid
Smooth muscle relaxants (mebeverine, alverine)	Inadequate evidence of safety – avoid
Tinidazole	Avoid in first trimester

Treatment of gastrointestinal symptoms and disease in lactation

Once the baby is delivered, its risk from treatment of gastrointestinal disease in the mother is mainly through the mother's milk in breastfeeding. Treatment should be in consultation between those providing postnatal care for the mother and the baby and the physician.

Although many drugs are secreted in the breast milk, they are not necessarily harmful to the baby, particularly if the minimum effective dose is used and the course is short. Prescribing requires intelligent and well-informed balancing of the risks of ingestion of the drug in breast milk against the benefits of continued breastfeeding for the baby and the mother. Table 5.2

lists drugs used in the treatment of gastrointestinal conditions that are secreted in breast milk, and indicates any special precautions needed.

Table 5.2: Commonly prescribed drugs for the treatment of gastrointestinal disease in lactation.

Drugs	Safety in lactation
Azathioprine	Avoid
5-ASA derivatives (sulphasalazine, mesalazine, olsalazine)	Small concentrations excreted in breast milk – probably safe
Cisapride	Avoid due to risk of prolonged QT interval in infant
Corticosteroids	Small concentrations present in breast milk – may be used
Domperidone	Low secretion – probably safe
H$_2$-receptor antagonists (cimetidine, famotidine, nizatidine, ranitidine)	Small concentrations present in breast milk – may be used
Interferon	Limited transfer into breast milk. Inadequate safety data – avoid
Proton pump inhibitors (omeprazole, lanzoprazole, pantoprazole)	Absorption in infant likely to be minimal. Inadequate safety data
Mebeverine	Low secretion – probably safe
Metoclopramide	Small concentrations present in breast milk – may be used
Metronidazole	Avoid large single doses
Octreotide	Avoid
Ranitidine bismuth citrate	Avoid

References

1 Fagan EA (1995) Disorders of the gastrointestinal tract. In *Medical Disorders in Obstetric Practice* (3rd edn) (ed M de Swiet), pp. 379–422. Blackwell Science, Oxford.

2 Magee LA, Inocencion G, Kamboj L *et al.* (1996) Safety of first-trimester exposure to histamine H$_2$ blockers. *Digest Dis Sci.* **41**(6): 1145–9.

3 Lalkin A, Loebstein R, Addis A *et al.* (1998) The safety of omeprazole during pregnancy: a multi-center prospective controlled study. *Am J Obstet Gynaecol.* **179**(3, Pt 1): 727–30.

4 Källén B (1998) Delivery outcome after the use of acid-suppressing drugs in early pregnancy, with special reference to omeprazole. *Br J Obstet Gynaecol.* **105**: 877–81.

5 Fagan EA (1995) Disorders of the liver, biliary system and pancreas. In *Medical Disorders in Obstetric Practice* (3rd edn) (ed M de Swiet), pp. 321–78. Blackwell Science, Oxford.

6 Fagan EA (1996) Liver and gastrointestinal disease in pregnancy. In *Oxford Textbook of Medicine* (3rd edn) (eds DJ Weatherall, JGG Ledingham and DA Warrell), pp. 1796–803. Oxford University Press, Oxford.

7 Lewis JH and Weingold AB (1985) The use of gastrointestinal drugs during pregnancy and lactation. *Am J Gastroenterol.* **80**: 912–23.

8 Atlay RD and Weekes AR (1986) The treatment of gastrointestinal disease in pregnancy. *Clin Obstet Gynaecol.* **13**: 335–47.

9 Whitelaw A and Butterfield A (1977) High breast milk sodium in cystic fibrosis. *Lancet.* **ii**: 1288.

10 Korelitz BI (1985) Pregnancy, fertility and inflammatory bowel disease. *Am J Gastroenterol.* **80**(5): 365–70.

11 Zeldis JB (1989) Pregnancy and inflamatory bowel disease. *West J Med.* **151**: 168–71.

12 Donaldson RM (1985) Management of medical problems in pregnancy: inflammatory bowel disease. *N Eng J Med.* **312**(25): 1616–19.

13 Hudson M, Flett G, Sinclair TS *et al.* (1997) Fertility and pregnancy in inflammatory bowel disease. *Int J Gynae Obstet.* **58**: 229–37.

14 Khosla R and Willoughby CP (1984) Crohn's disease and pregnancy. *Gut.* **25**: 52–6.

15 Fraser FC and Sajoo A (1995) Teratogenic potential of corticosteroids in humans. *Teratology.* **51**: 45–6.

16 Bell CM and Habal FM (1997) Safety of topical 5-aminosalicylic acid in pregnancy. *Am J Gastroenterol.* **92**(12): 2201–2.

17 Diav-Citrin O, Park YH, Veerasuntharam G *et al.* (1998) The safety of mesalamine in human pregnancy: a prospective controlled cohort study. *Gastroenterology.* **114**: 23–8.

18 Alstead EM, Ritchie JK, Lennard-Jones JE *et al.* (1990) Safety of azathioprine in pregnancy in inflammatory bowel disease. *Gastroenterology.* **99**: 443–6.

19 Reyes MP, Ostrea EM, Cabinian AE *et al.* (1989) Vancomycin during pregnancy: does it cause hearing loss or nephrotoxicity in the infant? *Am J Obstet Gynecol.* **161**(4): 977–81.

20 Witter FR, King TM and Blake DA (1981) The effects of chronic gastrointestinal medication on the fetus and neonate. *Obstet Gynecol.* **58**(Suppl 5): 79S–84S.

CHAPTER SIX

Hypertension

Martin Parkinson

Introduction

As a group, hypertensive disorders are the most common potentially serious problem in pregnancy, affecting 10–15% of pregnancies. They are a major cause of maternal death in the UK and the most common cause of prematurity. Hypertension accounts for up to 25% of antenatal admissions and much of antenatal care, especially in the second half of pregnancy, is aimed at the detection of hypertension and pre-eclampsia.[1,2]

Cardiac output increases during pregnancy and peripheral resistance falls, so that the maternal blood pressure falls in the first trimester, reaches a nadir in the second trimester and returns to pre-pregnancy levels in the third trimester. The possible aetiologies of hypertension in pregnancy are shown in Box 6.1. The first two clinical presentations are often mixed, leading to the concept of pre-eclampsia superimposed on underlying chronic hypertension.

Box 6.1: Hypertensive disorders during pregnancy[2]

- Hypertension caused by pregnancy:
  - pregnancy-induced hypertension (PIH)
  - pre-eclampsia: a specific disorder of pregnancy characterised by hypertension and proteinuria.
- Chronic hypertension (revealed during pregnancy but not due to pregnancy).

Definition

Chronic hypertension may be present before, or begin during, pregnancy. A diastolic blood pressure above 90 mmHg before 20 weeks gestation suggests chronic hypertension. Firm evidence is not available on the optimal threshold for treatment. However, there is consensus that treatment is essential at ≥170/100 mmHg. Mild to moderate chronic hypertension (140–169/90–109 mmHg) is unlikely to be dangerous for mother or fetus and drug treatment should be withheld until after delivery, although there is much variation in individual clinical practice with many treating at ≥140/90 mmHg. However, the risk of progression to pre-eclampsia[3] necessitates that these women are closely monitored.

Most complications are related to superimposed pre-eclampsia, which leads to a significantly higher incidence of intrauterine growth retardation (IUGR), premature delivery, Caesarean section, placental abruption and increased perinatal mortality.[4] Pre-eclampsia is highly dangerous for both mother and fetus and requires immediate hospital management.

If hypertension is diagnosed for the first time in pregnancy, secondary causes such as renal disease, phaeochromocytoma or coarctation of the aorta should be excluded. The optic fundi and cardiovascular system should be examined, including palpation for radiofemoral delay and auscultation of the abdomen for renal artery bruits. Renal disease is the most important underlying factor. Renal function and urinalysis should be carried out. A plasma creatinine value of more than 100 micromol/L is abnormal during pregnancy. Endocrine causes are much rarer. It is important to consider autoimmunity, especially the antiphospholipid antibody syndrome, which has serious implications for the long-term health of the woman and the success of the pregnancy. The antiphospholipid antibody syndrome increases the risk of miscarriage, of IUGR and of early-onset pre-eclampsia.[5]

Superimposed pre-eclampsia is detected by frequent monitoring of blood pressure and urine, serial measurements of plasma urate (hyperuricaemia is indicative of impaired renal tubular function) and a platelet count (looking for an abnormal fall) in the second half of pregnancy.[5] The frequency of monitoring needs to be tailored to the individual, but should be at least every two weeks from the 24th week onwards. High-risk women should preferably be monitored in a specialist clinic.

Hypertension which develops after the 20th week of pregnancy in the absence of proteinuria is often referred to as pregnancy-induced hypertension (PIH). Pregnancy-induced hypertension has been defined as a single diastolic reading of 110 mmHg or greater, or two readings of 90 mmHg or greater at least four hours apart, occurring in a previously normotensive patient.[6]

Management

The aims of antihypertensive treatment during pregnancy are to protect the mother from cardiovascular complications and cerebral haemorrhage, without conveying risks to the fetus.[1,5] There are two main problems with the use of antihypertensives in pregnancy: (i) the potential teratogenic effects of most antihypertensives are unclear as very few studies have included women in the first trimester; consequently, the choice of drug in early pregnancy is restricted;[7,8] (ii) antihypertensives may also reduce placental blood flow which could lead to intrauterine growth retardation.

Treatment of mild to moderate hypertension (diastolic pressure below 110 mmHg) is of no benefit to the fetus[9,10] and does not prevent progression to severe hypertension or pre-eclampsia.* In general, therefore, levels below this should not be treated. Antihypertensive therapy should only be considered in severe hypertension.

The management of hypertension in women of child-bearing potential should reflect the lack of experience with most antihypertensives in early pregnancy. Women with pre-existing hypertension should be aware that their medication may be changed or stopped if they plan to become pregnant. In mild to moderate hypertension, treatment should preferably be stopped before, or as soon as possible after, conception unless there are compelling indications. If a woman is primigravid she should be aware that her risk of pre-eclampsia is increased and that her pregnancy will be closely monitored. There is no evidence that pregnancy worsens long-term hypertension. Treatment should always be reviewed at the end of the first trimester as blood pressure naturally falls at this time.

Methyldopa

Methyldopa is the antihypertensive of choice in pregnancy even though it is no longer first line in non-pregnant patients. Possible adverse effects include drowsiness and diarrhoea but these are generally transient. Depression can occur rarely, so it is probably best avoided in women with a history of depression. Methyldopa has been used extensively in pregnancy. A postulated association with reduced fetal head circumference[11] is of doubtful clinical

---

*In the case of mild to moderate pre-eclampsia there is some suggestion of a reduction in the risk of respiratory distress syndrome in infants born to such mothers. In addition, treatment has been shown to reduce the risk of progressing to severe hypertension in women with mild to moderate chronic hypertension, pregnancy-induced hypertension or pre-eclampsia, and reduces the incidence of proteinuria at the time of delivery in women with pregnancy-induced hypertension.[7]

importance; no effect on intellect or development has been found in follow-up of exposed children to eight years of age.[12] An overview of studies involving over 600 women concluded that methyldopa reduces the risk of developing severe hypertension but not that of developing pre-eclampsia.[13] It also revealed a trend towards a reduction in perinatal death. However, despite the review's conclusion, there is a lack of evidence to draw *firm* conclusions.

Beta-adrenoceptor blockers

There is little experience with beta-blockers in the first trimester but no evidence that they cause fetal malformations. Numerous studies have shown that they may reduce placental blood flow, reducing the supply of nutrients and oxygen to the baby and causing intrauterine growth retardation (IUGR).[14-16]* These effects are more likely if they are used during periods of rapid fetal growth in the second and particularly the third trimester. Comparative studies have shown differences in the potential of various beta-blockers to cause IUGR. Atenolol, metoprolol, pindolol and propranolol have all been associated with IUGR. The combined alpha- and beta-blocker, labetalol, has theoretical advantages over these agents and most randomised controlled trials have not detected IUGR.[17] Labetalol is widely used by obstetricians in the UK.

The use of beta-blockers in late pregnancy is associated with neonatal hypoglycaemia and bradycardia[14] and prolonged labour. If beta-blockers are used in late pregnancy they should, where possible, be stopped a few days before delivery. An overview of randomised controlled trials of beta-adrenoceptor blockers concluded that beta-blockers reduce the risk of severe hypertension, but not the risk of pre-eclampsia. Too few patients have been studied to allow reliable conclusions regarding their effects on neonatal morbidity or perinatal death.[18]

Calcium channel blockers

Published data on the effects of calcium channel blockers in pregnancy, especially in the first trimester, are limited but there is no evidence of teratogenic effects.[19,20] Most experience is with nifedipine for acute or long-term control of hypertension.[21] It is a useful second-line drug in women uncontrolled by methyldopa. It has a shorter half-life in pregnancy so should be administered as a modified release formulation.[22] It frequently causes headache, and flushing and dizziness may also occur.

---

*These studies are of poor quality and there is continued uncertainty about the risk of IUGR due to these agents.

Angiotensin-converting enzyme inhibitors

All angiotensin-converting enzyme (ACE) inhibitors are contraindicated. Exposure in early pregnancy appears not to be associated with congenital abnormalities[23] but in later pregnancy there may be a number of complications. ACE inhibitors decrease fetal renal function and urine production which can lead to a decrease in amniotic fluid volume (oligohydramnios).[24] Because the protective effect of amniotic fluid is removed, the uterus can then come into direct contact with the developing bones of the fetus, causing structural defects. Oligohydramnios may also lead to pulmonary hypoplasia, possibly resulting in fetal death. There are several reported cases of, occasionally irreversible, fetal renal failure resulting from *in utero* exposure to ACE inhibitors;[24] dialysis has sometimes been necessary soon after delivery.

Angiotensin II receptor antagonists

This is a new class of drugs; losartan was the first to be launched in the UK but others are now available. There is very little experience with these drugs in human pregnancy. Animal studies have shown serious problems, which are likely to be due to the effects of these agents on the renin–angiotensin–aldosterone system. These drugs should not be used in pregnancy.

Diuretics

Diuretics should be avoided during pregnancy because of their potential to interfere with the physiological expansion of plasma volume during pregnancy.[25] They are contraindicated in pre-eclampsia and IUGR where uteroplacental perfusion is already reduced. A meta-analysis of nine randomised trials involving more than 7000 women showed a reduced incidence of pre-eclampsia and a decreased tendency to have oedema or hypertension, although no benefit was shown on fetal outcome.[26]

Breastfeeding

Most antihypertensives are safe in breastfeeding (Table 6.1). No adverse effects have been reported with calcium channel blockers, methyldopa or ACE inhibitors.[27] Beta-adrenoceptor blockers can rarely cause symptoms of beta-blockade in the baby. Atenolol taken by a mother caused bradycardia, hypotension and cyanosis in a day-old baby.[28] Thiazide diuretics may theoretically decrease or inhibit milk production, but are unlikely to cause problems in the infant.[29]

Table 6.1:   Safety of antihypertensives in pregnancy and lactation

Drug	Stage of pregnancy	Safety in pregnancy	Safety in breastfeeding
Recommended			
Methyldopa	1st, 2nd and 3rd trimesters	No evidence of teratogenicity or adverse effects despite widespread use.	Safe.
Use with caution			
Beta-blockers (labetalol oxprenolol, pindolol)	1st trimester	Limited data. No evidence of teratogenicity.	Generally regarded as safe.
	2nd trimester	No evidence of adverse effects.	Propranolol, metoprolol, labetalol preferred.
	3rd trimester	Possible IUGR, neonatal hypoglycaemia and bradycardia.	Some risk of accumulation with water-soluble drugs (e.g. atenolol, acebutolol) and neonatal bradycardia has been reported.
Calcium channel blockers	1st and 2nd trimester	Limited data. No evidence of teratogenicity.	Small amounts excreted in milk. Probably safe.
	3rd trimester	May inhibit or delay labour.	
Hydralazine	1st and 2nd trimester	Limited data. No evidence of teratogenicity.	Limited data. Other agents preferred.
	3rd trimester	Single case report of possible lupus-like syndrome in mother and baby.	
Avoid			
Diuretics	1st, 2nd and 3rd trimester	May interfere with plasma volume expansion.	Probably safe.
Angiotensin-converting enzyme inhibitors (e.g. captopril, enalapril) and angiotensin II receptor antagonists	1st trimester	No evidence of increased risk of specific birth defects.	ACE inhibitors – amounts excreted too small to be harmful.
	2nd and 3rd trimester	**Contraindicated.** May cause oligohydramnios, structural fetal abnormalities, pulmonary hypoplasia and fetal death.	Angiotensin II antagonists – lack of data. Avoid.

Pre-eclampsia

Pre-eclampsia is unique to pregnancy and is the major cause of maternal death in the UK. It is believed to result from placental dysfunction leading to the release of substances into the maternal circulation that cause vascular endothelial dysfunction.[30] Primigravidae are 15 times more likely to develop pre-eclampsia than parous women. Women affected in their first pregnancy have a slightly lower chance of recurrence in subsequent pregnancies. The risk increases slightly with age. Predisposing factors include chronic hypertension, change of partner and a previous or family history of pre-eclampsia. Predisposing fetal factors include multiple pregnancy, hydatidiform mole and hydrops fetalis.[1] The only cure is delivery of the fetus.

Criteria for the diagnosis of pre-eclampsia include: a rise in diastolic blood pressure of >15 mmHg or >30 mmHg systolic from early pregnancy; or diastolic blood pressure >90 mmHg on two occasions four hours apart; or >110 mmHg on one occasion and proteinuria. The fetus is at risk from placental insufficiency, IUGR, asphyxia and placental abruption.[31,32]

Mild pre-eclampsia is usually associated with few maternal risks provided delivery is expedited. In its most severe form, however, it may cause renal failure, clotting disturbance, liver failure and uncontrolled hypertension leading to cerebral haemorrhage. Delivery must occur more urgently if severe manifestations develop. Symptoms such as abdominal pain and nausea due to stretching of the liver capsule, and those suggestive of cerebral and retinal oedema (headaches and seeing flashing lights), are ominous features. HELLP syndrome (**H**aemolytic anaemia, **E**levated **L**iver function tests and **L**ow **P**latelet counts) and renal failure are serious complications.

Pre-eclampsia may progress to eclampsia with little or no warning. Eclampsia is defined as the occurrence of a generalised seizure in pregnancy associated with hypertension and proteinuria. Convulsions may occur without warning but may be preceded by headache, visual disturbances, epigastric pain and hyper-reflexia.

Prevention

Many agents have been studied in the prevention of pre-eclampsia.[33] Diuretics, fish oils and calcium supplements have no clear benefits and cannot be recommended. Both antiplatelet agents and anticoagulants have been investigated. Studies with warfarin and heparin have shown no clear benefits and since both have potentially serious adverse effects they should not be used in an attempt to prevent pre-eclampsia.[34] Low-dose aspirin has been studied on the premise that thromboxane inhibition may prevent or reverse the underlying vasodilator/vasoconstrictor imbalance. Results of all studies, including CLASP, suggest that the incidence of pre-eclampsia is reduced by about a quarter.[35,36] However, aspirin did not significantly affect the incidence of proteinuria, eclampsia, IUGR, stillbirths or neonatal deaths. Routine prophylactic use of aspirin in all women perceived to be at risk of pre-eclampsia is therefore not justified. It is now recommended only in women with a history of severe, early onset pre-eclampsia in a previous pregnancy.[37,38] Aspirin 75 mg daily should be started at about 12 weeks gestation.

Recent research has suggested that a pathological state of oxidative stress may have a role in the development of pre-eclampsia. A randomised trial of supplementation with Vitamins C and E in 283 women at 16–22 weeks' gestation was associated with a marked decrease in the frequency of pre-eclampsia.[39] These findings need to be confirmed in larger numbers of patients.

Management

Women who may have pre-eclampsia should be admitted to hospital for further investigation of maternal and fetal well-being, management of hypertension and planning of the delivery. Hydralazine, labetalol and nifedipine are the preferred antihypertensives for acute, severe pre-eclampsia.[2,17,40] Predicting if an individual woman will develop eclampsia is difficult; studies suggest that seizures occur in only 1–3% of women with severe pre-eclampsia. In Europe, IV diazepam or phenytoin was preferred for the treatment and prevention of eclampsia until recently, while magnesium sulphate was used in the United States. Magnesium sulphate is now known to be superior to diazepam and phenytoin in the prevention of recurrent seizures and is the anticonvulsant of choice.[41]

Summary

- All primigravida and any woman at risk should have their blood pressure measured and urine checked for protein fortnightly from 24 weeks gestation then weekly closer to term (certainly from 36 weeks).[42]
- Women with some degree of hypertension but no proteinuria need expert assessment and frequent monitoring but not necessarily admission.
- Hospital admission is usually indicated if proteinuria is also present (Box 6.2). Excessive weight gain, thrombocytopenia, hyperuricaemia, raised liver enzymes or evidence of intrauterine growth retardation point to pre-eclampsia and favour admission.

Box 6.2:   Indications for hospital admission

Admit on the same day:

- women with proteinuria ('1+' or more) in the presence of hypertension (diastolic 90 mmHg or more)
- women with blood pressure greater than 160/100 mmHg whether or not proteinuria is present.

Admit as an emergency:

- women with hypertension, proteinuria and symptoms (headache, visual disturbance, epigastric pain or nausea).

References

1   Redman C (1995) In *Hypertension in Pregnancy: Medical disorders in obstetric practice* (3rd edn) (ed M de Swiet). Blackwell Scientific, Oxford.

2   Redman CWG (1994) Hypertension in pregnancy. In *Textbook of Hypertension* (ed JD Swales). Blackwell Scientific, Oxford.

3   Rey E and Couturier A (1994) The prognosis of pregnancy in women with chronic hypertension. *Am J Obstet Gynecol.* **171**: 410–16.

4   Sibai BM and Anderson GD (1986) Pregnancy outcome of intensive therapy in severe hypertension in first trimester. *Obstet Gynecol.* **67**: 517–22.

5   Teoh TG and Redman CW (1996) Management of pre-existing disorders in pregnancy: hypertension. *Prescrib J.* **36**(1): 28–36.

6   Davey DA and MacGillivray I (1988) The classification and definition of the hypertensive disorders of pregnancy. *Am J Obstet Gynecol.* **158**: 892–8.

7   Magee LA, Ornstein MP and von Dadelszen P (1999) Management of hypertension in pregnancy. *BMJ.* **318**: 1332–6.

8   Gallery EDM (1995) Hypertension in pregnancy. Practical management recommendations. *Drugs.* **49**(4): 555–62.

9   Sibai BM, Mabie WC, Shamsa F *et al.* (1990) A comparison of no medication versus methyldopa or labetalol in chronic hypertension during pregnancy. *Am J Obstet Gynecol.* **162**: 960–7.

10   Redman CWG (1991) Controlled trials of antihypertensive drugs in pregnancy. *Am J Kid Dis.* **17**: 149–53.

11   Moar VA, Jefferies MA, Mutch LMM *et al.* (1978) Neonatal head circumference and the treatment of maternal hypertension. *Br J Obstet Gynaecol.* **85**: 933–7.

12   Cockburn J, Moar VA, Ounstead M *et al.* (1982) Final report of a study on hypertension during pregnancy: the effects of specific treatment on the growth and development of children. *Lancet.* **i**: 647.

13   Collins R and Wallenburg HCS (1995) In *Effective Care in Pregnancy and Childbirth* (eds I Chalmers, M Enkin and M Kierse). Oxford University Press, Oxford.

14   Eliahou HE, Silverberg DS, Reisin E *et al.* (1978) Propranolol for the treatment of hypertension in pregnancy. *Br J Obstet Gynaecol.* **85**: 431.

15 Pruyn SC, Phelan JP and Buchanan GC (1979) Long-term propranolol therapy in pregnancy: maternal and fetal outcome. *Am J Obstet Gynecol.* **135**: 485.

16 Butters L, Kennedy S and Rubin C (1990) Atenolol in essential hypertension during pregnancy. *BMJ.* **301**: 587–9.

17 Rey E, LeLorier J, Burgess E *et al.* (1997) Report of the Canadian Hypertension Society Consensus Conference. 3. Pharmacological treatment of hypertensive disorders in pregnancy. *Can Med Assoc J.* **157**: 1245–54.

18 Collins R and Duley L (1995) Beta-blockers vs methyldopa in the treatment of pre-eclampsia. In *Oxford Database of Perinatal Trials* (ed I Chalmers). Update Software, Oxford.

19 Magee LA, Schick B, Donnenfeld AE *et al.* (1996) The safety of calcium channel blockers in human pregnancy: a prospective, multicentre cohort study. *Am J Obstet Gynecol.* **174**: 823–8.

20 Constantine G, Beevers DG, Reynolds AL *et al.* (1987) Nifedipine as a second-line antihypertensive drug in pregnancy. *Br J Obstet Gynaecol.* **94**: 1136–42.

21 Levin AC, Doering PL and Hatton RC (1994) Use of nifedipine in the hypertensive diseases of pregnancy. *Ann Pharmacother.* **28**(12): 1371–8.

22 Prevost RR, Aki SA, Whybrew WD *et al.* (1992) Oral nifedipine pharmacokinetics in pregnancy-induced hypertension. *Pharmacother.* **12**: 174–7.

23 Lip GYH, Churchill D, Beevers M *et al.* (1997) Angiotensin-converting enzyme inhibitors in early pregnancy. *Lancet.* **350**: 1446–7.

24 Hanssens M, Keirse MJ, Vankelecom F *et al.* (1991) Fetal and neonatal effects of treatment with angiotensin-converting enzyme inhibitors in pregnancy. *Obstet Gynecol.* **78**: 128–35.

25 Sibai BM, Grossman RA and Grossman HG (1984) Effects of diuretics on plasma volume in pregnancies with long-term hypertension. *Am J Obstet Gynecol.* **150**: 831–5.

26 Collins R, Yusuf F and Peto R (1985) Overview of randomised trials of diuretics in pregnancy. *BMJ.* **290**: 17–23.

27 Anderson PO (1991) Drug use during breastfeeding. *Clin Pharm.* **10**: 594–624.

28 Diamond JM (1989) Toxic effects of atenolol consumed during breastfeeding [letter]. *J Pediatr.* **115**(2): 336.

29 Tveite WP (1994) Drugs and breastfeeding: a risk/benefit evaluation. *Vet Hum Toxicol.* **36**(1): 1–80.

30 Redman CWG and Roberts JM (1993) Management of pre-eclampsia. *Lancet.* **341**: 1451–4.

31 MacGillivray I (1983) *Pre-eclampsia: the hypertensive disease of pregnancy.* WB Saunders Company Ltd, London.

32 Roberts JM and Redman CWG (1993) Pre-eclampsia: more than pregnancy-induced hypertension. *Lancet.* **341**: 1447–51.

33 Carroli G, Duley L, Belizan JM *et al.* (1994) Calcium supplementation during pregnancy: a systematic review of randomised controlled trials. *Br J Obstet Gynaecol.* **101**: 753–8.

34 The Cochrane Collection (1995) *Warfarin/heparin in pre-eclampsia. The Cochrane database of perinatal trials.* Update Software, Oxford.

35 CLASP (Collaborative Low-Dose Aspirin Study in Pregnancy) Collaborative Group (1994) CLASP: a randomised trial of low-dose aspirin for the prevention and treatment of pre-eclampsia among 9364 pregnant women. *Lancet.* **343**: 619–29.

36   Sibai BM, Caritis SN, Thom E *et al.* (1993) Prevention of pre-eclampsia with low-dose aspirin in healthy nulliparous pregnant women. *New Engl J Med.* **329**: 1213–18.

37   Darling M and Higgins J (1994) CLASP: millstone or milestone? [editorial]. *Lancet.* **343**: 616–7.

38   Duley L (1999) Aspirin for preventing and treating pre-eclampsia. *BMJ.* **318**: 751–2.

39   Chappell LC, Seed PT, Briley AL *et al.* (1999) Effects of antioxidants on the occurrence of pre-eclampsia in women at increased risk: a randomised trial. *Lancet.* **354**: 810–16.

40   Mushambi MC, Halligan AW and Williamson K (1996) Recent developments in the pathophysiology and management of pre-eclampsia. *Br J Anaesth.* **76**: 133–48.

41   Eclampsia Trial Collaborative Group (1995) Which anticonvulsant for women with eclampsia? Evidence from the Collaborative Eclampsia Trial. *Lancet.* **345**: 1455–63.

42   Managing high blood pressure in pregnancy (1993) *Drug Ther Bull.* **31**(14): 53–6.

CHAPTER SEVEN

Other cardiovascular disorders

Martin Parkinson

Thromboembolism

Pregnancy, and especially the post-partum state, are risk factors for venous thrombosis and pulmonary embolism. The incidence of deep vein thrombosis (DVT) during pregnancy may be as high as one in 200 deliveries and is higher post-partum.[1,2] Women undergoing Caesarean section are up to 16 times more likely to develop a DVT than those delivered vaginally. Pulmonary embolism is relatively less common, affecting one in 2000 pregnancies, but it remains one of the most common causes of maternal death.[3]

Anticoagulant therapy during pregnancy

The management of anticoagulation during pregnancy presents some particularly challenging problems.

Warfarin

Warfarin is a known human teratogen; its use during pregnancy can lead to a well recognised series of facial and skeletal abnormalities known as the fetal warfarin syndrome.[4–6] Nasal hypoplasia is the most consistent feature; the bridge of the nose is depressed, resulting in a flattened, upturned appearance. In addition there is often stippling of cartilage and soft tissues secondary to abnormal calcification, growth retardation and short extremities. Obstruction of the upper airways may lead to neonatal respiratory depression. Death in infancy is common. Less common features include eye defects, congenital heart disease and developmental retardation. The critical period of exposure seems to be between the sixth and ninth weeks of gestation; about 5–10% of fetuses exposed during this period will be affected.[4] Treatment at any time in the first trimester is associated with a spontaneous abortion rate of about 15%. Stillbirths and neonatal death may also occur.[7,8] The overall rate of adverse fetal outcome after warfarin exposure is probably about 16%.[9]

Since the period of susceptibility is in early pregnancy, at a time when many women may not realise that they are pregnant, it is extremely important that all women of child bearing potential taking anticoagulants are counselled about possible fetal risks. They must be advised not to become pregnant without first discussing it with their doctor.

Exposure to warfarin both before and after this period has been linked with other congenital abnormalities.[4,10,11] Central nervous system defects, possibly the result of haemorrhage and scarring and subsequent impaired brain tissue growth, may develop following exposure to warfarin during any stage of pregnancy. These include malformations of the optic pathway, corpus callosum agenesis, Dandy–Walker malformation, areas of atrophy, encephalocoeles, microcephaly and hydrocephalus. Sequelae of this damage include mental retardation, blindness, spasticity and epilepsy. Fetal haemorrhage during the second and third trimesters may also cause damage in previously normally formed organs. In addition, the use of warfarin late in pregnancy may result in bleeding complications for both mother and baby at delivery.[8] Fetal harm is not only linked with poor anticoagulant control, it can occur with good control.

Heparin

Heparin is the anticoagulant of choice in pregnancy as it does not cross the placenta.[5] Heparin (unfractionated) appears to be relatively safe for the fetus, but long-term therapy can cause maternal osteoporosis.[12] Most cases have been reported following administration of at least 15 000 units daily over a minimum of six months,[13,14] although one case has been reported after the use of 10 000 units daily for 36 weeks.[15] Heparin may cause thrombocytopenia in up to 5% of patients, usually after about a week's treatment. Platelet counts should therefore be monitored before, and at regular intervals during, treatment. Heparin use in late pregnancy may put the mother at risk from haemorrhage during delivery, although protamine may be used to reverse this if necessary.

Low-molecular-weight heparins

Studies have shown that low-molecular-weight heparins (LMWH), although containing shorter and lighter molecules than standard, unfractionated heparin, do not cross the placenta.[16–18] They have a number of potential advantages over standard heparin, particularly in obstetrics where prophylaxis is required over long periods of time. They have an increased bioavailability and half-life, allowing once-daily administration, and they have a more predictable dose–response relationship. In addition, the risk of thrombocytopenia is less[19] and there may be a lower risk of osteoporosis.[20] Although LMWHs are unlicensed for use in pregnancy, experience with their use is accumulating and published data suggest that they are a safe and effective alternative to standard heparin in obstetric thromboprophylaxis.[20–24]

Thrombolytics

The use of thrombolytic therapy during pregnancy is an extremely difficult issue requiring specialist advice. Generally, it should be reserved for those patients with life-threatening conditions such as pulmonary embolism or, in the extremely rare situation, myocardial infarction. It is absolutely contraindicated near the time of delivery due to the risk of neonatal haemorrhage.

Prophylaxis of thromboembolism

Thromboprophylaxis is advocated in pregnancy and the puerperium for women with previous recurrent thrombosis, women with inherited (protein C deficiency, protein S deficiency, antithrombin III deficiency and activated protein C resistance) and acquired (lupus anticoagulant or anticardiolipin antibodies) thrombophilia and women with a thromboembolic event in the current pregnancy.[2] Some obstetric units also offer heparin prophylaxis to women with a single previous thromboembolic event plus a family history of thromboembolism.[20] Low-risk women (who have had one previous episode of thromboembolism) should probably take low-dose aspirin (e.g. 75 mg daily) from as soon as pregnancy is confirmed until delivery.

Many prophylactic regimens have been advocated. In the past it was suggested that heparin should be used during the first 12 weeks of gestation, then replaced by warfarin until a few weeks before term when heparin would be restarted. Concern about the safety of warfarin at any stage of pregnancy has led to the currently preferred option of using only heparin throughout pregnancy.[25] Care must be taken to minimise the risk of osteopenia. Practice varies in different obstetric centres and local obstetric protocols should be consulted.

Unfractionated heparin is given subcutaneously to achieve levels (using the anti-factor Xa assay) of approximately 0.1 unit/mL throughout pregnancy. If heparin levels are not available, a dose of approximately 7000 units twice daily has been suggested. The international normalised ratio (INR) or prothrombin time should also be monitored regularly to ensure that the lowest effective doses are used and that haemorrhage is avoided.

Treatment of deep vein thrombosis

Treatment of established DVT in pregnancy entails special risks. Bed rest with leg elevation may provide some symptomatic relief and possibly reduce the chance of re-embolism. Anticoagulation with IV heparin is vital; a loading dose, similar to that used in non-pregnant patients, is given followed by a continuous infusion. The heparin dosage should be monitored closely and adjusted accordingly. Again, local obstetric protocols should be followed.

Thromboprophylaxis for mechanical heart valve prostheses

Box 7.1:   Thromboprophylaxis in women with prosthetic heart valves

- Patients require a high degree of anticoagulation.
- Heparin is the safest option.
- Some experts advocate warfarin use throughout pregnancy.
- Women must be counselled about the fetal risks before pregnancy.

Women with mechanical heart valve prostheses require a high level of anticoagulation in order to prevent valve thrombosis. This carries a significant risk of fetal harm and the best method of achieving a high level is controversial. It has been suggested that heparin prophylaxis may be insufficient to prevent valve thrombosis,[26–28] so some experts have advocated the use of warfarin throughout pregnancy. Consequently, cases of fetal warfarin embryopathy have appeared in the recent literature.[29] This is a difficult issue with regard to the balance of maternal and fetal risk, but heparin is clearly the safer treatment option for the fetus and warfarin should be avoided wherever possible. Low-molecular-weight heparin may be a useful treatment option for the future, but experience to date in this situation is extremely limited.[30] All women with prosthetic heart valves who wish to have children require careful pre-pregnancy counselling.

Treatment of arrhythmias

Cardiac arrhythmias may develop in otherwise healthy pregnant women, but frequently are associated with underlying acquired or congenital heart disease. Occasionally, paroxysmal atrial tachycardia, Wolff–Parkinson–White syndrome or both may increase in frequency during pregnancy. Arrhythmias may affect placental blood flow, possibly resulting in fetal harm. In general, the management of arrhythmias is unchanged in pregnancy. Indications for anticoagulation are unchanged; however, heparin, not warfarin, should be used.

The management of pregnant women with arrhythmias is highly specialised, requiring collaboration between GP, cardiologist and obstetrician. Safety considerations with anti-arrhythmic agents in pregnancy have recently been reviewed.[31,32]

Anticoagulants in breastfeeding

Warfarin is not contraindicated in breastfeeding. It is highly protein bound in the maternal circulation, therefore very little is secreted into milk.[33,34] There is no evidence that bleeding in the infant has occurred. Nevertheless, the baby should be observed for excessive bruising or petechiae.[35] Due to its high molecular weight, heparin is unlikely to transfer into milk; any reaching the milk would be rapidly destroyed in the infant's gut.

Hyperlipidaemia

Box 7.2:   Hyperlipidaemia

- Primary hyperlipidaemia is a long term condition probably not requiring drug treatment during pregnancy.
- There are few data on the effects of fibrates and statins on pregnancy so they should not be used.
- Cholestyramine is not absorbed from the gut. Fat-soluble vitamins, folic acid and iron supplements should be given if it is used in pregnancy.
- Lipid-regulating drugs should not be given to breastfeeding mothers.

Hyperlipidaemia is rare during pregnancy, but certain genetic conditions predispose to raised serum cholesterol levels possibly requiring treatment during pregnancy. However, in most cases therapy for hyperlipidaemia may be discontinued or withheld during pregnancy with little or no impact on the long-term outcome of hypercholesterolaemia.

Fibrates

There is no evidence that exposure to fibrates during pregnancy has adverse effects on the fetus, although there are insufficient data to recommend their use. Women exposed inadvertently during the first trimester may be reassured.

Cholestyramine

Cholestyramine is an anionic exchange resin which binds bile acids within the gut and the complex is then excreted in the faeces. Since cholestyramine is not absorbed, or susceptible to enzymatic hydrolysis within the gut, it is unlikely to have direct adverse effects on the fetus and the risks appear to be minimal. Cholestyramine has been used successfully during pregnancy to relieve pruritus induced by cholestasis. Since the resin effectively binds bile salts, lowering the bile-salt concentration in the intestinal lumen, the solubilisation and absorption of fat and fat products declines. Consequently, the absorption of fat-soluble vitamins (A, D, E and K) and possibly other nutrients such as folic acid and iron may be impaired. Although deficiencies in fat-soluble vitamins are uncommon, several cases have been reported. The administration of prenatal vitamin and mineral supplements two to three hours after a dose of cholestyramine would alleviate this potential problem.

HMG-CoA reductase inhibitors

There are few data on the effects of hydroxy-methylglutaryl co-enzyme A (HMG-CoA) reductase inhibitors in human pregnancy (e.g. simvastatin and pravastatin). Products of the cholesterol biosynthesis pathway are essential to fetal development, therefore there are theoretical reasons not to use them during pregnancy. This is supported by animal experiments in which an association was found between inhibition of cholesterol biosynthesis at the same step as the statins and fetal malformations. Although limited data do not suggest that statins are teratogenic when inadvertently used during the first trimester,[36] there are insufficient data to recommend their use during pregnancy.

Lipid-regulating drugs in breastfeeding

There is a lack of data on the safety of all these drugs in breastfeeding. Cholestyramine is not secreted into breast milk. The effects of exposure to fibrates and statins via breast milk are unknown. However, as cholesterol and other products of cholesterol biosynthesis are essential for neonatal development, these drugs should not be given to mothers who are breastfeeding.[35]

References

1   de Swiet M (ed) (1995) Thromboembolism. In *Medical Disorders in Obstetric Practice* (3rd edn). Blackwell Scientific, Oxford.
2   Royal College of Obstetricians and Gynaecologists (1995) *Thromboembolic Disease in Gynaecology and Pregnancy: recommendations for prophylaxis.* RCOG, London.
3   Department of Health, Welsh Office, Scottish Home and Health Department and Department of Health and Social Services, Northern Ireland (1996) *Confidential Enquiries into Maternal Deaths in the United Kingdom 1991–1993.* The Stationery Office, London.
4   Hall JG, Pauli RM and Wilson KM (1980) Maternal and fetal sequelae of anticoagulation during pregnancy. *Am J Med.* **68**: 122–40.
5   Ginsberg JS, Hirsh J, Turner DC *et al.* (1989) Risks to the fetus of anticoagulant therapy during pregnancy. *Thromb Haemostas.* **61**(2): 197–203.
6   Greaves M (1993) Anticoagulants in pregnancy. *Pharm Ther.* **59**: 311–27.
7   Ginsberg JS and Hirsh J (1988) Optimum use of anticoagulants in pregnancy. *Drugs.* **36**: 505–12.
8   Ginsberg JS and Hirsh J (1998) Use of antithrombotic agents during pregnancy. *Chest.* **114**: S524–S530.
9   Frewin R and Chrisholm M (1998) Anticoagulation of women with prosthetic heart valves during pregnancy. *Br J Obstet Gynaecol.* **105**: 683–6.
10   Kaplan LC and Anderson GG (1982) Congenital hydrocephalus and Dandy–Walker malformation associated with warfarin use during pregnancy. *Birth Def.* **18**: 79.
11   Barbour LA and Pickard J (1995) Controversies in thromboembolic disease during pregnancy: a critical review. *Obstet Gynaecol.* **86**(4): 621–33.
12   Griffith GC, Nichols G, Asher JD *et al.* (1965) Heparin osteoporosis. *JAMA.* **193**: 92–4.
13   Haram K, Hervig T, Thordarson H *et al.* (1993) Osteopenia caused by heparin treatment in pregnancy. *Obstet Gynaecol Scand.* **72**: 674–5.
14   de Swiet M (1992) Selected side-effects: Heparin and osteoporosis. *Prescrib J.* **32**(2): 74–7.
15   Dahlman TC (1993) Osteoporotic fractures and the recurrence of thromboembolism during pregnancy and the puerperium in 184 women undergoing thromboprophylaxis with heparin. *Am J Obstet Gynecol.* **168**: 1265–70.
16   Forestier F, Sole Y, Aiach M *et al.* (1992) Absence of transplacental passage of fragmin (Kabi) during the second and the third trimesters of pregnancy. *Thromb Haemostas.* **67**(1): 180–1.
17   Omri A, Delaloye JF, Andersen H *et al.* Low-molecular-weight heparin Novo (LHN-1) does not cross the placenta during the second trimester of pregnancy. *Thromb Haemostas.* **61**(1): 55–6.

18   Fejgin MD and Lourwood DL (1994) Low-molecular-weight heparins and their use in obstetrics and gynecology. *Obstet Gynecol Surv*. **49**(6): 424–31.

19   Warkentin TE, Levine MN, Hirsh J *et al*. (1995) Heparin-induced thrombocytopenia in patients treated with low-molecular-weight heparin or unfractionated heparin. *N Engl J Med*. **332**: 1330–5.

20   Nelson-Piercy C, Letsky EA and de Swiet M (1997) Low-molecular-weight heparin for obstetric thromboprophylasis: experience of 69 pregnancies in 61 women at high risk. *Am J Obstet Gynecol*. **176**(5): 1062–8.

21   Gillis S, Shushan A and Eldor A (1992) Use of low-molecular-weight heparin for prophylaxis and treatment of thromboembolism in pregnancy. *Int J Gynaecol Obstet*. **39**: 297–301.

22   Dulitzki M, Pauzner R, Langevitz P *et al*. (1996) Low-molecular-weight heparin during pregnancy and delivery: preliminary experience with 41 pregnancies. *Obstet Gynecol*. **87**: 380–3.

23   Hunt BJ, Doughty HA, Majumdar G *et al*. (1997) Thromboprophylaxis with low-molecular-weight heparin (Fragmin) in high-risk pregnancies. *Thromb Haemostas*. **77**: 39–43.

24   Sturridge F, Letsky EA and de Swiet M (1994) The use of low-molecular-weight heparin for thromboprophylaxis in pregnancy. *Br J Obstet Gynaecol*. **101**: 69–71.

25   Greer IA and de Swiet M (1993) Thrombosis prophylaxis in obstetrics and gynaecology. *Br J Obstet Gynaecol*. **100**: 37–40.

26   Iturbe-Alessio I, del Carmen Fonseca M, Mutchinik O *et al*. (1986) Risks of anticoagulant therapy in pregnant women with artificial heart valves. *N Engl J Med*. **315**: 1390–3.

27   Hanania G, Thomas D, Michel PL *et al*. (1994) Pregnancy and prosthetic heart valves: a French cooperative retrospective study of 155 cases. *Eur Heart J*. **15**: 1651–8.

28   Wang RYC, Lee PK, Chow JF *et al*. (1983) Efficacy of low-dose, subcutaneously administered heparin in treatment of pregnant women with artificial heart valves. *Med J Aust*. **2**: 126–7.

29   Wellesley D, Moore I, Heard M *et al*. (1998) Two cases of warfarin embryopathy: a re-emergence of this condition? *Br J Obstet Gynaecol*. **105**: 805–6.

30   Lee LH, Liauw PCY and Ng ASH (1996) Low-molecular-weight heparin for thromboprophylaxis during pregnancy in two patients with mechanical mitral valve replacement. *Thromb Haemostas*. **76**: 627–31.

31   Chow T, Galvin J and McGovern B (1998) Anti-arrhythmic drug therapy in pregnancy and lactation. *Am J Cardiol*. **82**(4A): 581–621.

32   Jose AJ and Page RL (1999) Treatment of cardiac arrhythmias during pregnancy. *Drug Safety*. **20**(1): 85–94.

33   Orme ML'E, Lewis PJ, de Swiet M *et al*. (1977) May mothers given warfarin breastfeed their infants? *BMJ*. **1**: 1564–5.

34   McKenna R, Cole ER and Vasan U (1983) Is warfarin sodium contraindicated in the lactating mother? *J Pediatr*. **103**: 325–7.

35   Hale TW (1998) *Medications and Mothers' Milk*. Pharmasoft Medical Publishing, Amarillo, Texas.

36   Manson JM, Freyssinges C, Ducrocq MB *et al*. (1996) Post-marketing surveillance of lovastatin and simvastatin exposure during pregnancy. *Reprod Toxicol*. **10**(6): 439–46.

CHAPTER EIGHT

Respiratory disorders

Steve Chaplin

Asthma

Pregnancy

Asthma is the most common respiratory disorder occurring during pregnancy, affecting about 5% of women of child-bearing age. The prevalence of asthma in pregnancy has been reported to be 1% but this is likely to be a substantial underestimate.[1]

Studies investigating the effect of pregnancy on asthma are conflicting but there appears to be no consistent effect on asthma morbidity:[1-3]

- there is no change in one-third to one-half of women
- asthma improves in about a third of cases
- it gets worse in one-quarter to one-third.

Knowing the history of previous pregnancies is often useful because the course and outcome of a current pregnancy will be similar in about two-thirds of women. However, there is a substantial minority of women in whom the effects of pregnancy on asthma are unpredictable and potentially troublesome. It is therefore important to monitor symptoms and lung function closely and to adjust treatment. As the British Thoracic Society (BTS) guidelines for the management of asthma in adults emphasise,[4] treatment may need to be stepped up or down. Ideally, treatment will be optimised before conception, with the aim of establishing prophylaxis and symptom control with the least potential risk to the fetus. Women of child-bearing age with asthma should therefore be advised to consult their GP when planning a family.

Severe asthma has been associated with adverse fetal outcome, including an increased risk of pre-term labour and low birth weight.[5-9] These associations may be due to chronic, or intermittent, maternal hypoxaemia and may not accurately reflect the risk for milder disease or its treatment. The effects of uncontrolled asthma are undoubtedly serious: severe exacerbations cause fetal hypoxia and a severe asthma attack is potentially fatal for the mother and fetus.[2]

The drug treatment of asthma in pregnancy is essentially the same as in the non-pregnant woman (Table 8.1). In general, the main classes of drugs used are thought to be safe for the fetus.[10] These drug classes have been widely used without evidence of significant risk and are therefore the drugs of choice:

short-acting bronchodilators:	salbutamol, terbutaline
inhaled corticosteroid:	beclomethasone, budesonide
oral steroid:	prednisolone
prophylactic medications:	cromoglycate.

Table 8.1: Drug treatment of asthma in pregnancy and lactation

Class	Drug	Pregnancy	Breastfeeding
Short-acting bronchodilators (inhaled)	Salbutamol, terbutaline and other short-acting selective beta$_2$-agonists	Negligible risk to fetus Fenoterol has more marked cardiovascular activity and is best avoided Inhalation is the preferred route	Negligible risk
Short-acting bronchodilators (oral)	Salbutamol Terbutaline	At high doses, risk of fetal tachycardia, hyperkalaemia Impaired glucose control in women with diabetes	Concentration of terbutaline negligible
Long-acting bronchodilator	Salmeterol	Risk uncertain due to relatively limited use	Risk uncertain due to relatively limited use
Corticosteroids (inhaled)	Beclomethasone Budesonide Fluticasone	Negligible risk to fetus Most experience with beclomethasone Risk with fluticasone uncertain due to relatively limited use Inhalation is the preferred route	Negligible risk

Table 8.1: continued

Class	Drug	Pregnancy	Breastfeeding
Corticosteroids (oral)	Prednisolone	Prednisolone is the oral steroid of choice Risk of cleft palate in animal studies, not substantiated in humans Prolonged exposure may cause fetal adrenal suppression, but this is rarely clinically important	> 40 mg/day prednisolone or equivalent may cause adrenal suppression
Theophyllines	Aminophylline Theophylline	Theophylline clearance increased during pregnancy Neonatal toxicity reported (apnoea, irritability)	Risk of adverse effects at high maternal blood concentrations. Modified-release formulations preferred
Other anti-inflammatory agents	Cromoglycate Nedocromil	Apparently low risk Risk with nedocromil uncertain due to relatively limited use	Negligible risk
Anticholinergic agents	Ipratropium Oxitropium	Apparently low risk with ipratropium Risk with oxitropium uncertain due to relatively limited use	Uncertain. but systemic levels after inhalation probably negligible
Leukotriene receptor antagonists	Montelukast Zafirlukast	Lack of data – avoid	Lack of data – avoid

Bronchodilators

Beta$_2$-agonists are effective bronchodilators and have been the mainstay of asthma therapy for decades. Inhaled bronchodilators are preferred. Studies have shown no adverse pregnancy outcome in women who used inhaled beta-agonists in the first trimester.[11] There is limited experience with oral bronchodilators in pregnancy and they may have the potential to inhibit labour during later pregnancy. Experience with longer-acting bronchodilators such as salmeterol, fenoterol and eformoterol is limited and these agents should preferably be avoided unless control cannot be achieved with other agents.

Antimuscarinic bronchodilators

Ipratropium or oxitropium may be used by inhalation in the management of chronic asthma in patients who already require high-dose inhaled corticosteroids. These should be used with caution in pregnancy as there is very little published data on their use. However, there is no evidence that antimuscarinic agents are associated with increased fetal risk.

Theophylline

Theophylline may be introduced at step three or four of the BTS asthma guidelines. Modified release preparations may be particularly useful in controlling nocturnal symptoms. Some studies have postulated that theophylline may be associated with fetal harm, but this requires confirmation.[12,13] It may be used with caution in pregnant women.

Corticosteroids

Studies in animals have demonstrated teratogenicity (particularly cleft palate but also reduced birthweight) with high doses of corticosteroids. However, these effects appear to be species-specific and have not been supported by convincing evidence in humans.[14,15] When administered for prolonged periods during pregnancy, systemic corticosteroids significantly increase the risk of intrauterine growth retardation.[15] There is a theoretical risk of adrenal suppression in the neonate following prenatal corticosteroid exposure. However, this usually resolves spontaneously after birth and is rarely clinically important.

It is difficult to distinguish the possible risk of drug therapy from that of asthma because a controlled study (in which the controls are women with untreated asthma) cannot be carried out. Studies in women with asthma treated with oral or inhaled steroids have provided evidence of a good outcome (although some lack controls).[6,16]

One recent comparison of pregnancy outcome in 486 women with asthma with that in healthy controls[17] found only a significant relationship between oral corticosteroid use (associated with severe asthma) and pre-eclampsia, but even this was of dubious importance because the incidence of pre-eclampsia was unusually low in controls and the statistical significance became borderline after controlling for maternal hypertension. An increase in low-birth-weight children associated with oral corticosteroids was not statistically significant. Other drugs used by women in this study included inhaled bronchodilators, theophylline, cromoglycate and inhaled steroids. This study confirms the findings of earlier studies in similar groups of women.

In a recent study investigating the effect of an acute asthma attack in pregnancy, it was found that the risks of an attack were higher in women with inadequate inhaled anti-inflammatory treatment.[18] It is important that women do not stop using their inhaled corticosteroids due to anxiety about their effects on the fetus.

Other medications

Sodium cromoglycate may be used during pregnancy as there is no evidence of increased fetal risk.[10] The new leukotriene inhibitors montelukast and zafirlukast are given orally. There is no published experience with these drugs in human pregnancy so their use cannot be recommended.

Management during labour

Asthma rarely complicates labour, perhaps due to increased endogenous production of glucocorticoids and catecholamines.[2] Management of an acute attack during labour is the same as at any other time with immediate administration of a beta$_2$-agonist bronchodilator. However, earlier use of steroids is indicated if the initial response is unsatisfactory. Drugs which may cause bronchospasm should be used with caution during labour; examples include prostaglandins and ergometrine.

Regional anaesthesia is preferable to general anaesthesia because of the risk of a chest infection secondary to atelectasis. There is a risk of bronchoconstriction with pethidine and other opioids but effective analgesia should not be withheld.

Breastfeeding

Blood concentrations of bronchodilators and corticosteroids are very low after inhalation and pose little risk to the neonate. Theophylline does occur in breast milk but the concentrations associated with the use of modified-release formulations (which avoid high maternal blood levels and account for virtually all theophylline preparations now in use) are low and probably unimportant. Prednisolone reaches breast milk in small amounts. However, doses of up to 40 mg of prednisolone daily are unlikely to cause systemic effects in the infant.[15] Women should be encouraged to breastfeed because of the benefits to the baby, particularly in terms of reducing the risk of atopic disease.

In summary, the drugs used to treat asthma pose little or no risk during pregnancy or while breastfeeding. By contrast, the risks of poorly controlled asthma are severe. The principles of management are therefore unchanged, although the BTS guidelines do not appear to have been formally evaluated in pregnant women. In fact, since these guidelines emphasise the importance of monitoring, prophylaxis and minimising drug doses, they should be followed closely. In particular, inhalation is preferable to oral administration because maternal blood levels – and therefore fetal doses – are substantially lower, especially during high-dose steroid treatment. Women should be involved in the management of their asthma and education should be provided to ensure they understand the importance of good control during pregnancy.

Allergic rhinitis

Pregnancy

The management of allergic rhinitis (including perennial rhinitis and hay fever) presents a dilemma: the symptoms are unpleasant for the sufferer but rarely debilitating, so do the benefits of drug treatment justify the potential risk to the fetus? The options include oral and intranasal antihistamines, intranasal corticosteroids and oral and intranasal decongestants (Table 8.2). There is a lack of evidence on which to base recommendations but a pragmatic approach would be:

- avoid drugs during the first trimester if possible
- choose intranasal over oral administration (making steroids the drugs of choice)
- avoid sympathomimetic decongestants when possible.

Table 8.2: Drug treatment of allergic rhinitis in pregnancy and lactation

Class	Drug	Pregnancy	Breastfeeding
Antihistamines	Chlorpheniramine	Long experience implies risk very low	May occur in milk; risk uncertain. Clemastine associated with drowsiness in infant
	Brompheniramine	Limited evidence suggests some risk; safety therefore uncertain	
	Terfenadine	No evidence of risk but use limited compared with chlorpheniramine	
	Astemizole	Avoid (defects reported in animals); no longer available in the UK	
Corticosteroids	Beclomethasone Betamethasone Budesonide Flunisolide Fluticasone	Risk probably negligible with intranasal use	Risk probably negligible with intranasal use
Cromoglycate	Sodium cromoglycate	Risk probably negligible with intranasal use	Risk probably negligible with intranasal use
Decongestants	Pseudoephedrine Phenylephrine Phenyl-propanolamine Oxymetazoline Xylometazoline	Limited evidence of risk but relevance to intermittent use for rhinitis unclear Pharmacological effects on fetus possible with oral use Excessive intranasal use associated with significant systemic absorption	Pseudoephedrine not present in significant concentrations; risk with other agents uncertain

The risks of antihistamines appear to be low.[21] The sedating antihistamine chlorpheniramine has been used for many years with no evidence of teratogenicity in man, including use specifically for morning sickness. There is some doubt about brompheniramine, for which the American Collaborative Perinatal Project[22] found a statistically significant association with congenital malformations, but good supporting evidence is lacking. Caution suggests that an older antihistamine should be used in preference to newer agents, though the risk of drowsiness may make this impracticable. The newer but widely used terfenadine has the advantage of being non-sedating; there is no evidence suggesting it is associated with malformations but its safety is unconfirmed.[23] High doses of astemizole (now discontinued in the UK) are associated with defects in animals and the manufacturer recommends avoidance during pregnancy. The frequency of congenital anomalies was not increased among 104 infants whose mothers had taken astemizole in the first trimester in a cohort study.[24] Astemizole has a long half-life and patients are advised to avoid conception for several weeks after the last dose.

The safety of other, newer antihistamines is also unconfirmed though some are active metabolites of long-established, sedating antihistamines (for example, cetirizine is a metabolite of hydroxyzine).[25] A recent prospective controlled study in 92 women exposed to either hydroxyzine or cetirizine found no evidence of an increased teratogenic risk. Most antihistamines are available from pharmacies without prescription; the packaging normally carries a warning against use during pregnancy but this is more to encourage women to consult the GP than because of a significant risk to the fetus.

In principle, it is preferable to choose an intranasal antihistamine such as azelastine since this would produce lower maternal blood concentrations. However, intranasal use is less effective than oral administration against symptoms affecting the eyes and is probably less effective than intranasal steroids against nasal symptoms.

There are several steroids for intranasal use formulated as sprays (beclomethasone, budesonide, flunisolide, fluticasone) or drops (betamethasone). Beclomethasone is available from pharmacies without prescription. These are probably the agents of choice for prophylaxis, particularly when symptoms affect only the nose. Intranasal cromoglycate is an alternative but it is believed to be less effective than a topical steroid. None of these agents are likely to pose a significant risk during pregnancy.

Decongestants are sympathomimetics and may cause tachycardia and transient increases in blood pressure in the mother, and presumably affect the fetus too. Statistical associations with minor malformations have been reported[22] but there is a lack of clear evidence that the intermittent administration characteristic of their use in rhinitis is associated with abnormalities. Excessive use of intranasal formulations is associated with significant systemic absorption and symptoms in adults, although the risk during pregnancy is unknown. Since intranasal decongestants may be associated with rebound hyperaemia, encouraging repeated use, they are probably best avoided. Some over-the-counter formulations contain a combination of sympathomimetics and antihistamines.

Breastfeeding[19,20]

The drugs of choice for breastfeeding women are intranasal steroids which give rise to negligible concentrations in milk. Antihistamines may occur in significant levels; whether these are sufficient to affect the infant is uncertain but drowsiness has been associated with clemastine which is marketed specifically for the relief of hay fever.[26] The sympathomimetic pseudoephedrine does not occur in milk in pharmacologically significant levels.

References

1   Moore-Gillon J (1994) Asthma in pregnancy. *Br J Obstet Gynecol.* **101**: 658–60.
2   de Swiet M (ed) (1995) Diseases of the respiratory system. In *Medical Disorders in Obstetric Practice* (3rd edn), pp. 1–47. Blackwell Scientific, Oxford
3   Greenberger PA (1992) Asthma in pregnancy. *Clin Chest Med.* **13**(4): 597–605.
4   Ayres, JG, Barnes PJ, Bellamy D *et al.* (1997) *The British Guidelines on Asthma Management: 1995 review and position statement. Thorax.* **52**(Suppl 1): S20–S21.
5   Bahna SL and Bjerkedal T (1972) The course and outcome of pregnancy in women with bronchial asthma. *Acta Allergol.* **27**: 397–400.
6   Fitzsimmons R, Greenberger PA and Patterson R (1986) Outcome of pregnancy in women requiring corticosteroids for severe asthma. *J Aller Clin Immunol.* **78**: 349–53.
7   Doucette JT and Bracken MB (1993) Possible role of asthma in the risk of pre-term labour and delivery. *Epidemiology.* **4**: 143–50.
8   Schatz M, Zeiger RS and Hoffman CP (1990) Intrauterine growth is related to gestational pulmonary function in pregnant asthmatic women. Kaiser-Permanente asthma and pregnancy study group. *Chest.* **98**: 389–92.
9   Kramer MS, Coates AL, Michoud MC *et al.* (1995) Maternal asthma and idiopathic pre-term labour. *Am J Epidemiol.* **142**: 1078–88.
10   Schatz M (1997) Asthma treatment during pregnancy: what can be safely taken? *Drug Safety.* **16**(5): 342–50.
11   Mabie WC (1996) Asthma in pregnancy. *Clin Obstet Gynecol.* **39**(1): 56–69.
12   Park JM, Schmer U and Myers TL (1990) Cardiovascular anomalies associated with prenatal exposure to theophylline. *South Med J.* **83**: 1487–8.
13   Briggs GG, Freeman RK and Yaffe SJ (1994) *Drugs in Pregnancy and Lactation: a reference guide to fetal and neonatal risk* (4th edn). Williams and Wilkins, Baltimore.
14   Fraser FC and Sajoo A (1995) Teratogenic potential of corticosteroids in humans. *Teratology.* **51**: 45–6.
15   CSM/MCA (1998) Systemic corticosteroids in pregnancy and lactation. *Current Problems in Pharmacovigilance.* **24**: 9.
16   Greenberger PA and Patterson R (1983) Beclomethasone dipropionate for severe asthma during pregnancy. *Ann Intern Med.* **98**: 478–80.
17   Schatz M, Zeiger RS, Hoffman CP *et al.* (1995) Perinatal outcomes in the pregnancies of asthmatic women: a prospective controlled analysis. *Am J Resp Crit Care Med.* **151**: 1170–4.
18   Stenius-Aarniala BSM, Hedman J and Teramo KA (1996) Acute asthma during pregnancy. *Thorax.* **51**: 411–14.

19   Hale T (1998) *Medications and Mothers' Milk* (7th edn). Pharmasoft Medical Publishing, Amarillo, Texas.

20   Bennett PN (1996) *Drugs and Human Lactation* (2nd edn). Elsevier, Amsterdam.

21   Schatz M, Zeiger RS, Harden K *et al.* (1997) The safety of asthma and allergy medications during pregnancy. *J Aller Clin Immunol.* **100**: 301–6.

22   Heinonen OP, Sloane D and Shapiro S (1977) *Birth Defects and Drugs in Pregnancy*, pp. 323–4. Publishing Sciences Group, Littleton, Massachusetts.

23   Schick B, Hom M, Librizzi R *et al.* (1994) Terfenadine exposure in early pregnancy. *Teratology.* **49**(5): 417.

24   Pastuszak A, Schick B, D'Alimonte D *et al.* (1996) The safety of astemizole in pregnancy. *J Aller Clin Immunol.* **98**: 748–50.

25   Einarson A, Bailey B, Jung G *et al.* (1997) Prospective controlled study of hydroxyzine and cetirizine in pregnancy. *Ann Aller Asthma Immunol.* **78**(2): 183–6.

26   Kok THHG, Taitz LS, Bennett MJ *et al.* (1982) Drowsiness due to clemastine transmitted in breast milk. *Lancet.* **1**: 914–5.

CHAPTER NINE

Epilepsy

Susanna Gilmour-White

Epilepsy is the most common major neurological disorder encountered by obstetricians, with one in 200 pregnancies occurring in women with epilepsy. Concerns these women may have include the worry that pregnancy will increase the risk of seizures, the effect of seizures on the pregnancy and fetus and whether medication will cause malformations in the child. The management of epilepsy in pregnancy is difficult as most anti-epileptic drugs have known teratogenic effects. However, in most cases women can be reassured that pregnancy will be unaffected and that there is a more than 90% chance of a normal infant.[1]

This chapter covers the choice of contraception, the risks and benefits of drug treatment, drug level monitoring, and the use of folic acid and vitamin K. It highlights the need for forward planning and for addressing anxieties before pregnancy occurs, especially as epilepsy affects all aspects of pregnancy. The management of a woman with epilepsy wishing to conceive can be divided into four stages:

1 pre-conception
2 during pregnancy
3 delivery
4 after the birth.

Pre-conception

Young women with epilepsy should be aware that pregnancy carries some additional risks for them as soon as they become sexually active. They should be urged to seek medical advice before a planned pregnancy. Ideally, the management of pregnancy in these women requires collaboration between GP, obstetrician and neurologist or epilepsy specialist.

Contraception in women taking anti-epileptic medication

Combined oral contraceptive pill (COC)

Some anti-epileptic drugs interact with oral contraceptives, but despite this combined oral contraceptives can be used by most women.

In the majority of women a contraceptive pill containing at least 20 µg of oestrogen is needed to inhibit ovulation. The most widely prescribed oral contraceptives contain 30 µg, for example Microgynon 30, Eugynon 30, Ovran 30 and Ovranette all contain 30 µg ethinyloestrodiol.

The anti-epileptic drugs which induce liver enzymes, carbamazepine, phenytoin, phenobarbitone, primidone and topiramate, increase the rate of metabolism of both oestrogens and progestogens and this may lower blood concentrations to levels at which they are ineffective.[2] Sodium valproate, lamotrigine, vigabatrin and gabapentin do not affect the metabolism of the contraceptive pill. Women taking an enzyme-inducing anti-epileptic drug who wish to take a COC should take a pill or pills that contain at least 50 µg of oestrogen. Although this can be done simply with Ovran, other possibilities include a double dose of a 30 µg pill or a combination of a 20 µg and a 30 µg oestrogen pill, which gives greater flexibility where higher doses are needed.

An alternative regime that may be useful in some women is the three monthly or 'tricycle' system. In this, the chosen pill(s) is taken for three cycles continuously before a shorter than normal break of five days. This is thought to give greater protection than the standard 21-day regime. It is thought that the pill-free interval is a time of risk in some women, and this risk is increased by drug interactions affecting pill hormone levels.[4] Women with epilepsy taking enzyme-inducing anti-epileptic drugs fit into this group.

Some women, or their doctors, may be concerned about the risks of high doses of oral oestrogen; however, this is unfounded. In the presence of induced enzymes these doses result in oestrogen levels comparable to those achieved with 30 µg preparations.[3]

Breakthrough bleeding indicates that contraception cannot be assured and that a larger dose of oestrogen is needed. However, even a regular menstrual cycle without breakthrough bleeding cannot always be taken as a totally reliable guide. If ovulation has taken place the blood progesterone concentration normally rises tenfold by day 21. This measurement will confirm whether or not ovulation has been inhibited and can be done reliably on day 21 of a cycle where the pill was started on day one to three (as recommended), but the test will have to wait until the second cycle if the pill is started later.

Progesterone-only pill (POP)

Progestogens are also affected by enzyme inducing anti-epileptic medication which may lead to breakthrough bleeding. Furthermore, progesterone-only pills require rigorous compliance. If, however, these are chosen, women should take at least double the dose.

Intramuscular medroxyprogesterone (Depo-Provera)

Intramuscular medroxyprogesterone (Depo-Provera) is a possible alternative in women who have difficulty remembering to take daily medicine. It is metabolised almost completely on a single pass through the liver so that liver enzyme induction has little impact. In fact, clearance of this drug is more dependent on the liver blood flow than liver enzyme activity. Interactions with enzyme-inducing drugs are therefore not a problem.[5]

Pre-conceptional treatment review

This is an opportunity to review the diagnosis, the need for continued anti-epileptic treatment, the possibility of changing to a single drug or changing the preparation. At this stage the advice of an epilepsy specialist should be sought.

Hereditary factors

The known inherited/genetic conditions associated with epilepsy can be divided broadly into two groups. The first, the inherited/genetic epilepsies, include benign familial neonatal or infantile convulsions and familial frontal lobe epilepsy. Many of this group are autosomal dominant, which implies a risk of up to 50% of transmitting the gene to offspring.[6]

The second group is the inherited neurological conditions in which epilepsy may occur, for example Down's syndrome and tuberous sclerosis. These diseases usually present in childhood and are normally clinically evident before child-bearing age.

If these conditions are excluded, however, then the risk of a mother with epilepsy having an affected child is approximately 5%; the same risk if both parents are normal but have a previously affected child. The risk rises to 10% if one parent and one older sibling have epilepsy.[7]

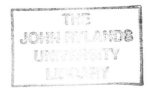

Therapeutic issues

Fertility and miscarriage

Anti-epileptic drugs are not thought to cause infertility in women and this includes the four newer drugs – vigabatrin, lamotrigine, gabapentin and topiramate – so far as is known. Some drugs may affect male fertility, and this has been ascribed to altered sperm motility and reduced circulating testosterone concentrations, but the data are insubstantial.[8] There is some suggestion that men and women with epilepsy may be less fertile than the general population, even without medication.[9,10] The risk of miscarriage is not increased by epilepsy or anti-epileptic drugs.[11]

Teratogenicity

There is extensive literature on the use of anti-epileptic drugs during pregnancy. Much of this is contradictory, but it is known that all the commonly used drugs carry a teratogenic risk. The incidence of serious malformations in the offspring of the general population is about 2–3%. This rises to about 4% in women with epilepsy and, if anti-epileptic drugs are taken, to about 5%. Abnormalities are more likely if the mother takes more than one anti-epileptic drug; evidence suggests an incidence of about 10% with three drugs and 20% with four.[12–14] However, women taking several anti-epileptics are likely to have more severe epilepsy which may account in part for the observed increased risk.

The problems seen most frequently are minor dysmorphic anomalies affecting the face and digits (Box 9.1). These have been described with all the main anti-epileptics. Factors involved are thought to include genetic predisposition and the severity of the maternal trait of epilepsy. With the exception of hypertelorism, many of the other features become less apparent as the child grows. Major abnormalities (Box 9.2) can also be attributed to all traditional drugs, especially when used in combination, but occur less frequently. Whether each drug can cause a specific fetal 'syndrome' is debatable since there is a great deal of overlap between the patterns of abnormalities described.

Box 9.1:   Minor abnormalities

- V-shaped eyebrows
- Low-set ears
- Broad nasal bridge
- Irregular teeth or wide mouth
- Hypertelorism (a wider than normal space between the eyes)
- Hypoplasia of the nails and distal phalanges

Box 9.2:   Major abnormalities

* Orofacial clefts
* Congenital heart disease (septal defects)
* Neural tube defects

The data relating to effects on growth or intellectual development, although fairly extensive, provide limited information. Excluding the obvious malformations, lasting effects in the majority of children appear to be minimal.[15]

Animal studies suggest that teratogenic risk is correlated with high doses of anti-epileptic drugs. This association has not been established conclusively in human studies so far, except with sodium valproate and spina bifida.[16,17] In general, if good control is achieved on a single drug there is little to be gained by switching to a drug perceived to be associated with a lower risk.[18]

Phenytoin

Phenytoin may cause minor defects in up to 30% of exposed infants.[19] A characteristic pattern of malformations termed 'fetal hydantoin syndrome' has been described, comprising craniofacial and digital defects, intellectual deficiency and intrauterine growth retardation. However, similar anomalies have been described in babies born to women with epilepsy not exposed to phenytoin. Phenytoin is associated with an increased incidence of heart defects and cleft palate of 1.8% compared with 0.7% in the general population.[20]

Sodium valproate

Sodium valproate is known to increase the risk of neural tube defects. Exposure during the critical period of gestation (days 17 to 30 after fertilisation) carries a 1–2% risk of neural tube defects. This risk is about the same as for a familial recurrence of the disorder, which is about 50 times higher than the rate in the general population (0.023%).[21] Risk is correlated with the dose of valproate used.

Where valproate is considered necessary for a woman who is pregnant or is planning a pregnancy, the risks may be minimised by keeping the dose as low as possible, giving the daily dose in divided doses and considering the use of modified-release preparations which will avoid high-peak serum concentrations. The existence of a specific fetal valproate syndrome has been suggested but many of the abnormalities described are similar to those seen with anti-epileptic drugs in general.[22]

Carbamazepine

Until recently, carbamazepine was felt to be relatively safe in pregnancy. However, in 1991 an association with neural tube defects was reported.[23] The risk of this defect is thought to be about 0.5–1%.

Newer drugs (lamotrigine, vigabatrin, gabapentin, topiramate, tiagabine)

Very little is known about the risks of the newer anti-epileptics.[24] In animal studies vigabatrin and topiramate have shown some teratogenicity.[25] Lamotrigine is a weak inhibitor of dihydrofolate reductase and consequently carries a theoretical risk of neural tube defects. Gabapentin has not shown teratogenicity in animals.

Experience of these drugs in human pregnancy is extremely limited. Vigabatrin has already been implicated in some cases of congenital malformations. For the present, while so little is known about them, these drugs should not be used unless absolutely necessary. Moreover, these newer drugs are likely to be given as part of 'combination therapy', with its possible attendant risks. The British Neurological Surveillance Unit is currently compiling a register of women exposed to these drugs.

Suspected adverse effects of any drug used during pregnancy should be reported to the Committee of Safety of Medicines through the 'yellow card' scheme. Some pharmaceutical manufacturers have data on pregnancy outcome after exposure to their drugs which is usually available on request. The company may ask for details of the pregnancy in question in order to expand their database.

Folic acid

The Department of Health encourages all women contemplating pregnancy to eat folate-rich foods and to take a 400 µg folic acid supplement until the 12th week of pregnancy (*see* Chapter 13). Women who have had a previous child with a neural tube defect are advised to take 5 mg daily for the same period.[26] Carbamazepine and sodium valproate are associated with an increased risk of neural tube defects. Folate deficiency may also be implicated in some of the facial malformations associated with phenytoin.[27] Moreover, although ambiguous, results of other work speculate a link between orofacial clefts and folic acid unrelated to anti-epileptics.[28] These data add weight to the opinion of most experts that women with epilepsy should take 5 mg folic acid per day at least for the first 12 weeks of pregnancy, regardless of the anti-epileptic they are taking.[29,30]

There are now several commercial preparations of 400 µg that can be prescribed or bought 'over the counter', but 5 mg tablets require a prescription. The folic acid supplement should be started from the time a woman stops contraception.

During pregnancy

Drug level monitoring

It is helpful to have the baseline blood levels of any anti-epileptic taken at the beginning of pregnancy. It is also wise to measure the serum albumin. Seizure frequency is increased in a third of women, a number of these may be due to reduced blood levels of the anti-epileptic. Poor compliance may follow anxiety about possible effects of the drug on the fetus and sickness may lead to malabsorption. The most important reasons for blood level changes, however, are due to pregnancy itself. Total anti-epileptic drug plasma concentrations may fall despite a constant oral dose. Factors involved include increased clearance by the maternal liver, increased plasma volume and a fall in albumin concentration which leads to decreased protein binding.

In women with well-controlled epilepsy, the fall in drug concentrations seldom causes problems. However, if epilepsy is poorly controlled, an increase in seizures is more likely. In these women the dose may be increased to maintain the blood level, but care should be taken. For example, during pregnancy the serum albumin can fall by as much as 30% and there may be an additional decrease in the binding capacity. These changes, affecting highly protein-bound drugs such as phenytoin, result in an increase of free active drug, although total drug levels may be unchanged or even low.[31,32]

The best practice is to adjust doses according to the woman's clinical condition, responding to seizure frequency rather than blood anti-epileptic levels. Some clinicians measure levels at constant intervals (every three to four months). This allows rapid dose adjustment to restore levels should seizures occur. If a dose increase has been necessary, it is important to adjust this back to the pre-pregnancy dose in the first few weeks after delivery.

Vomiting

If the problem is worst in the morning, anti-epileptic drugs that can be taken once daily, such as phenytoin or primidone, can be taken at night. Others, including carbamazepine and sodium valproate, that require twice or more daily dosing, could have the morning dose postponed for a few hours.

Investigations

The most important investigation in all women taking anti-epileptic drugs, particularly those on carbamazepine or sodium valproate, is high-definition ultrasound scanning early in the second trimester to exclude anencephaly and at 16–18 weeks to exclude spina bifida. This will also allow identification of cleft lip and palate and cardiac abnormalities. A rise in the maternal fetoprotein at 16 weeks has been used as an indicator of neural tube defects, but is not very reliable and aminiocentesis carries a 1% risk of miscarriage.

Effects of fits on the fetus

Minor fits appear to have no effect on the fetus. Major seizures associated with cyanosis, however, can lead to hypoxia and lactic acidosis in the infant. Falls resulting from fits can lead to trauma, early labour or miscarriage.

First fit in pregnancy

This is rare without obvious cause. These women should be referred for specialist neurological opinion about management and appropriate investigations.

In the second half of pregnancy diagnostic confusion can arise between a primary epileptic seizure or one associated with eclampsia. Urgent opinions from both neurological and obstetric specialties should be sought in this event.

Women with eclampsia will normally, though not always, have proteinuria at the time of the first fit. Other markers such as raised liver enzymes and creatinine concentration may be helpful in diagnosis.

Vitamin K

The enzyme-inducing anti-epileptic drugs (phenytoin, phenobarbitone, carbamazepine and topiramate) can cause vitamin K deficiency in the fetus. This may lead to deficiency in clotting factors and a risk of intracranial haemorrhage at birth. Although the mechanism remains unknown, there is evidence that placental transfer of vitamin K does occur from the mother to child.[33] Supplementation is strongly recommended.

There are several regimes for vitamin K supplementation in pregnant women taking anti-epileptic drugs. One example is to give the mother 20 mg vitamin K orally every day from 36 weeks, with 1 mg given IM to the baby on delivery.

Delivery

Delivery should be in hospital due to the risk of seizures during labour (about 1%). Most women have normal vaginal deliveries. Elective Caesarean section would be considered for those who have frequent generalised seizures during the later stages of pregnancy.

Some anti-epileptic drugs, particularly primidone, phenobarbitone and the benzodiazepines, are sedating and some infants show withdrawal symptoms in the first few days of life. Withdrawal fits are rare but most common with phenobarbitone.

After the birth

Breastfeeding

All of the established anti-epileptic drugs are excreted in breast milk. The list below shows the largest amount of drug likely to be received daily by an infant, expressed as a percentage of the recommended daily therapeutic dose for an infant:

- carbamazepine – 5%
- phenytoin – 5%
- sodium valproate – 3%
- phenobarbitone – 50%.

With the exception of phenobarbitone and primidone, mothers taking anti-epileptic drugs should be encouraged to breastfeed.

Of the newer drugs, lamotrigine, vigabatrin and gabapentin pass into breast milk in women, but there are no data on topiramate. Very little is known about their effects, if any, on breastfed babies. If the mother has been taking any one of these drugs during her pregnancy there seems little risk in breastfeeding the infant, with the exception of vigabatrin given its known risk of visual field defects. The amount of drug the baby would receive is likely to be small.

Post-partum contraception

Women should use contraception as soon as sexual activity is resumed. If hormonal contraception is used then it should be started 21 days post-delivery. The combined pill reduces milk supply, therefore progestogen-only pills should be taken by breastfeeding women who require an oral contraceptive. However, this is not ideal in women taking an enzyme inducing anti-epileptic drug and a non-hormonal method of contraception may be preferred until breastfeeding stops.

Review of anti-epileptic dose

Any increase in the dose of anti-epileptic therapy during pregnancy should be reviewed at this time. Blood levels of phenytoin increase rapidly after childbirth but the rebound in carbamazepine and sodium valproate is slower.

References

1   Delgado-Escueta AV and Janz D (1992) Consensus guidelines: pre-conception counselling, management and care of the pregnant woman with epilepsy. *Neurology.* **42**(5): 149–60.

2   Krauss GL, Brandt J, Campbell M *et al.* (1996) Anti-epileptic medication and oral contraceptive interactions: a national survey of neurologists and obstetricians. *Neurology.* **46**: 1534–9.

3   Orme M *et al.* (1991) Contraception, epilepsy and pharmacokinetics. In *Women and Epilepsy* (ed MR Trimble), pp. 145–58. Wiley, Chichester.

4   Guillebaud J (1993) *The Pill* (2nd edn). Oxford University Press, Oxford.

5   Association of the British Pharmaceutical Industry (1999) *Compendium of Data Sheets and Summaries of Product Characteristics 1999–2000.* Datapharm Publications, London.

6   Nashef L (1996) Definitions, aetologies and diagnosing. In *Treatment of Epilepsy* (2nd edn) (ed SD Shorvon). Blackwell Science, Cambridge, Massachusetts.

7   Harper PS (1988) *Practical Genetic Counselling* (3rd edn), p. 158. Wright, Bristol.

8   Dana-Haeri J, Oxley J and Richens A (1982) Reduction of free testosterone by anti-epileptic drugs. *BMJ.* **284**: 85–6.

9   Gautray JP, Jolivet A, Goldenberg F *et al.* (1978) Clinical investigation of the menstrual cycle. II. Neuroendocrine investigation and therapy of the inadequate luteal phase. *Fertil Steril.* **29**: 275–81.

10 Webber MP, Hauser WA, Ottman R *et al.* (1986) Fertility in persons with epilepsy. *Epilepsia.* **27**: 746–52.

11 Annegers JF, Baumgartner KB, Hauser WA *et al.* (1988) Epilepsy, anti-epileptic drugs and the risk of spontaneous abortion. *Epilepsia.* **28**: 451–88.

12 Lindhout D, Hoppener RJ, Meinardi H *et al.* (1984) Teratogenicity of anti-epileptic drug combinations with special emphasis on epoxidation (of carbamazepine). *Epilepsia.* **25**: 77–83.

13 Nakane Y, Okuma T, Takahashi R *et al.* (1980) Multi-institutional study on the teratogenicity and fetal toxicity of anti-epileptic drugs: a report of a collaborative study group in Japan. *Epilepsia.* **21**: 663–80.

14 Gaily E and Granstrom MJ (1989) A transient retardation of early postnatal growth in drug-exposed children of epileptic mothers. *Epilepsy Res.* **4**: 147–55.

15 Lindhout D *et al.* (1982) Hazards of fetal exposure to drug combinations. In *Epilepsy, Pregnancy and the Child: proceedings of a conference held 14–16 Sept, 1980 in West Berlin* (ed D Janz), pp. 275–81. Raven Press, New York.

16 Omtzigt JGC, Los FJ, Grobbee DE *et al.* (1992) The risk of spina bifida aperta after first-trimester exposure to valproate in a prenatal cohort. *Neurology.* **42**(5): 119–25.

17 Lindhout D, Omtzigt JG, Cornel MC *et al.* (1992) Spectrum of neural tube defects in 34 infants prenatally exposed to anti-epileptic drugs. *Neurology.* **42**(5): 111–18.

18   Delgado-Escueta AV and Janz D (1992) Consensus guidelines: pre-conception counselling, management and care of the pregnant woman with epilepsy. *Neurology.* **42**(5): 149–59.

19   Buehler BA, Delimont D, van Wiles M *et al.* (1990) Prenatal prediction of risk of the fetal hydantoin syndrome. *N Engl J Med.* **322**: 1567–72.

20   Perucca E and Richens A (1983) Anti-epileptic drugs, pregnancy and the newborn. In *Pharmacology and Obstetrics* (ed PJ Lewis), pp. 264–88. Wright, Bristol.

21   Lindhout D and Schmidt D (1986) *In utero* exposure to valproate and neural tube defects. *Lancet.* **iii**: 1392–3.

22   Clayton-Smith J and Donnai D (1995) Fetal valproate syndrome. *J Med Genet.* **32**: 724–7.

23   Rosa FW (1991) Spina bifida in infants of women treated with carbamazepine during pregnancy. *N Engl J Med.* **324**: 674–7.

24   Morrell MJ (1996) The new anti-epileptic drugs and women: efficacy, reproductive health, pregnancy and fetal outcome. *Epilepsia.* **37**(6): S34–S44.

25   Medical Information Departments of Hoechst Marion Russell (vigabatrin) and Janssen-Cilag (topiramate).

26   Department of Health, Letter, 18 December 1992. Addendum to CMO(92)18.

27   Biale Y and Lewenthal H (1984) Effect of folic acid supplementation on congenital malformations due to anticonvulsive drugs. *Eur J Obstet Gynecol Reprod Biol.* **18**: 211–16.

28   Shaw GM, Lammer EJ, Wasserman CR *et al.* (1996) Risks of orofacial clefts in children born to women using multivitamins containing folic acid preconceptually. *Lancet.* **346**: 393–6.

29   Duncan JS (1996) Reproductive aspects of epilepsy treatment. In *Treatment of Epilepsy* (2nd edn) (ed SD Shorvon). Blackwell Science, Cambridge, Massachusetts.

30   Cleland PG (1997) Management of pre-existing disorders in pregnancy: epilepsy. *Prescrib J.* **36**(2): 102–9.

31   Ruprah M, Perucca E, Richens A *et al.* (1980) Decreased serum protein binding of phenytoin in late pregnancy [letter]. *Lancet.* **2**: 316–17.

32   Ruprah M, Perucca E, Richens A *et al.* (1981) Phenytoin binding in pregnancy [letter]. *Lancet.* **1**: 97.

33   Thorp JA, Gaston L, Caspers DR *et al.* (1995) Current concepts and controversies in the use of Vitamin K. *Drugs.* **49**: 376–87.

Further reading

See also *Seizure* (1999) **8**: 201–17 which appeared just before this book went to press.

CHAPTER TEN

Psychiatric disorders

Alan James Worsley

Epidemiology

The psychiatric problems most often seen in pregnancy are depression and anxiety; psychosis occurs more rarely. Most pregnant women will experience some anxieties about the prospect of motherhood but these symptoms are not usually manifestations of an anxiety disorder. At least 10% of women will experience clinically significant anxiety during pregnancy[1] and this figure is probably higher in those who have had a previous termination or previous psychological illness.[2] During the puerperium about 10% of women become clinically depressed, a further 16% suffer from a self-limiting depressive episode and 0.2% of mothers develop psychotic illness.[3] Very few pregnant or puerperal women are referred to psychiatrists despite evidence that management of depression in these patients is sub-optimal.

Treatment

The management of pregnant women with a psychiatric disorder often requires the involvement of psychiatrist, obstetrician and general practitioner. Non-pharmacological treatments, such as cognitive and behavioural therapies, should be considered before resorting to drug therapy.

Where drug treatment is required, the benefits to mother and fetus must be weighed against the potential risks of no treatment. The risks of not treating may be high, for example if there is a risk of self-harm. Maternal psychiatric illness may also affect the future mother–child relationship. In women who conceive while taking psychotropic drugs there may be a significant risk of relapse if drug therapy is stopped.

There is a lack of good data on the risks of psychotropic therapy in pregnancy. Most studies suggest that these drugs are not associated with a significantly increased risk of birth defects. However, there is a risk of neonatal toxicity which may result in neonatal withdrawal symptoms and behavioural sequelae such as poor feeding and failure to thrive.

If drug treatment is given, an attempt should be made to use the lowest effective dose for the shortest period of time necessary, to minimise fetal exposure. However, it is acknowledged that for some drugs higher doses than those required by non-pregnant women may be needed to achieve symptom control, due to pharmacokinetic changes in pregnancy.

Depression

The prevalence of depression is about 8–10% in women of child-bearing age, although as few as a quarter of those who meet the criteria for major depression receive appropriate treatment.[4,5] Diagnosis in pregnancy can be complicated because symptoms such as fatigue, loss of energy and libido, and sleep disturbance, while consistent with depression, can occur normally at this time. Once diagnosed, the need for drug treatment will depend on symptom severity. If a woman with no previous history of depression develops symptoms during the first trimester, it is preferable to avoid medication unless symptoms are severe. If symptoms are moderate to severe, or if they persist after the first trimester, it is reasonable to treat.

In women taking an antidepressant who become pregnant or who wish to conceive, a trial of gradual drug withdrawal should be considered. However, if there is a history of recurrent moderate to severe depression, it is reasonable to continue treatment. Tricyclic and related antidepressants are the agents of choice, although selective serotonin re-uptake inhibitors (SSRIs) and related drugs may be used.

The risk of post-partum depression in women with a history of depression is about 25%.[6] Women with a history of severe post-partum depression may benefit from prophylactic antidepressants in the third trimester or the early puerperium. Although neonatal toxicity may occur due to antidepressant exposure in late pregnancy, this is often outweighed by the risks to the mother of stopping treatment before delivery.

Tricyclic antidepressants

Epidemiological studies of exposure to tricyclic antidepressants in pregnancy have not shown an increased risk of congenital malformations.[7] Despite early fears of an association with limb reduction defects,[8] no statistical increase in congenital anomalies has been detected in several large studies.[9–11] Outcome data after exposure to amitriptyline, imipramine and nortriptyline suggest that they are unlikely to have important teratogenic effects. Similar agents, including dothiepin, clomipramine and lofepramine, have all been used and although there are few outcome data there is no evidence that they are harmful.

Chronic use of high doses of tricyclic antidepressants, imipramine, amitriptyline and clomipramine near term has been associated with a neonatal withdrawal syndrome.[11-16] The neonatal withdrawal syndrome comprises symptoms such as irritability, tremulousness, diarrhoea, poor feeding, respiratory distress and seizures, normally occuring within 72 hours post-delivery. These symptoms may persist for several days or longer. Drugs associated with neonatal withdrawal include tricyclic antidepressants, SSRIs,[17-20] phenothiazines,[21,22] antihistamines,[23] opioids,[24-26] organic solvents,[27] alcohol[28] and benzodiazepines.[29-31] Neonatal withdrawal may occur with therapeutic doses but is more likely after the use of high doses and depot preparations.

Mild withdrawal symptoms in the neonate may be managed with non-pharmacological methods. Drug therapy may be required for more severe symptoms and pharmacological characteristics of the treatment options may be important. For example, chlorpromazine may be useful in neonatal withdrawal after phenothiazine exposure and phenobarbitone may be useful where seizures have occurred.

Standard doses of tricyclic and related drugs may be used to treat depression at any stage of pregnancy. Most experts recommend that the dose should be gradually reduced from about three to four weeks before the expected delivery date, to minimise the risk of neonatal withdrawal effects. However, the decision to do this depends on the mother's clinical condition and must take into account the risk of relapse.

Monoamine oxidase inhibitors

Data on the effects of monoamine oxidase inhibitors in human pregnancy are sparse. Animal data suggest possible teratogenicity.[32,33] The hypertensive reactions which can arise due to interactions with other medications and certain foods may have adverse effects on the fetus. Monoamine oxidase inhibitors are therefore not recommended in pregnancy.

Moclobemide

There are no published data on the use of moclobemide in human pregnancy and therefore its use cannot be recommended.

Selective serotonin re-uptake inhibitors and related drugs

As fluoxetine is now the most widely prescribed antidepressant worldwide, data on the effect of exposure in pregnancy are accumulating. There is no increase in the malformation rate of live-born infants.[34] It has been suggested in one study that there may be an increased rate of perinatal complications in women taking fluoxetine in the third trimester, including poor neonatal adaption, cyanosis on feeding and jitteriness.[35] However, other studies do not confirm that it is unsafe in pregnancy.[7,36]

There are few published data on the outcome of pregnancies exposed to paroxetine, sertraline, citalopram, fluvoxamine, venlafaxine, nefazadone, mirtazepine and reboxetine so their use in pregnancy cannot be supported.

In view of the relative lack of data on SSRIs, tricyclic antidepressants are the antidepressants of choice in pregnancy. If an SSRI is thought to be necessary then fluoxetine should be considered first.

If a woman becomes pregnant while taking a relatively new antidepressant, switching to another drug with more robust safety data should be considered, but is not always appropriate. In this situation, a psychiatric opinion would be valuable.

The serotonin re-uptake inhibitors, sertraline, fluoxetine and paroxetine, have been reported to cause neonatal withdrawal effects when used close to term.[17–20] If possible, the dose should be tapered from three to four weeks before the expected delivery date.

Tryptophan

Tryptophan, a natural precursor to serotonin, has been used together with other antidepressants. There are no data on its effects in pregnancy although it is unlikely to be harmful.

Electroconvulsive therapy (ECT)

Electroconvulsive therapy may be useful in depression when drugs are ineffective. It can produce rapid improvement in patients with severe depression accompanied with suicidal tendencies.[37] There is no evidence that ECT use during pregnancy is associated with an increased rate of miscarriage or other adverse fetal effects.[38–43]

Antidepressants and breastfeeding (Table 10.1)

Tricyclic antidepressants are excreted into breast milk. A small study of breastfeeding mothers treated with imipramine found no adverse effects in the infants.[44] Studies with amitriptyline and desipramine have not detected these drugs or their metabolites in the infant's serum.[45–49] It is thought to be safe for mothers taking tricyclic antidepressants to breastfeed. The infant should be monitored for sedation or irritability.

There are few data on the excretion of monoamine oxidase inhibitors (MAOIs) in breast milk. One study found tranylcypromine to be excreted into milk, but at levels not thought to be significant to the infant.[50] There are insufficient data available to recommend the use of traditional MAOI's in breastfeeding. Moclobemide, but not its active metabolite, has been detected in breast milk in small amounts considered unlikely to be a hazard to the infant.[51]

Data on the transfer of SSRIs to breast milk show that fluoxetine is excreted in relatively greater amounts than sertraline or paroxetine.[52] A single case report described severe colic, excessive crying and watery stools in an infant whose mother was taking 20 mg fluoxetine daily.[53] The symptoms disappeared when formula milk was given and recurred on rechallenge with breast milk. Available data for sertraline confirm that transfer into milk is minimal; no reports of adverse effects in nursing infants have been located. In general, sertraline or paroxetine would be a better choice of SSRI than fluoxetine for the breastfeeding mother.

There are no data on the deposition of tryptophan into breast milk although standard doses are unlikely to have adverse effects on the infant.

Table 10.1: Safety of antidepressants in pregnancy and lactation

Class	Drug	Pregnancy	Breastfeeding
Tricyclic and related drugs	Amitriptyline Imipramine Nortriptyline Clomipramine Dothiepin Lofepramine	Probably safe	Probably safe
	Mianserin Trazodone Doxepin	Limited outcome data – avoid	Avoid
SSRIs and related drugs	Fluoxetine	No evidence of increased fetal risk. May be used if tricyclic inappropriate	Use with caution
	Paroxetine Sertraline	Limited outcome data – avoid	Use with caution Preferable to fluoxetine

Table 10.1: continued

Class	Drug	Pregnancy	Breastfeeding
	Citalopram Nefazodone Venlafaxine Reboxetine	Limited outcome data – avoid	No data – avoid
MAOIs	Phenelzine	Limited outcome data – avoid	No data – avoid
Reversible MAOIs	Moclobemide	Limited outcome data – avoid	Lack of data – avoid

Key points

- For a first episode of depression arising during pregnancy, tricyclic antidepressants are the drugs of first choice.
- SSRIs and related drugs may be used where a tricyclic is inappropriate, e.g. where these are not tolerated or where there is a high risk of self-harm.
- In general, women with a history of depression should be treated with the drug which has been most effective previously. Medication throughout pregnancy is often warranted.
- In women taking an antidepressant who wish to become pregnant, it may be possible to withdraw therapy but a psychiatric opinion is advisable.

Manic (bipolar) disorders

Women previously diagnosed with bipolar illness are about three times more likely to have a relapse during pregnancy[54,55] and are at high risk for the development of post-partum psychosis. The usual treatment is prophylaxis with lithium, carbamazepine or sodium valproate, all of which are associated with specific fetal abnormalities. The main therapeutic issues are the risk of relapse or recurrence if prophylactic medication is withdrawn during pregnancy and the teratogenic potential of the medication.

It is vital that women who may become pregnant and are to be treated with lithium, carbamazepine or valproate receive adequate pre-conceptional counselling. They should be aware of the need for reliable contraception and the importance of seeking medical advice before a planned pregnancy. Management is likely to require close collaboration between general practitioner, obstetrician and psychiatrist. If possible, these drugs should be stopped during pregnancy, at least during the first trimester. The psychiatrist will be able to advise on whether this is possible and, if not, whether the dose of the medication may be reduced or the dosing frequency adjusted.

If it is possible to taper the dose of medication, this should be done slowly so not to precipitate relapse. If relapse occurs then medication should be resumed. A mother in a manic state may compromise her own safety and that of her child.

Carbamazepine

Most data on carbamazepine in pregnancy relate to its use in epilepsy (*see* Chapter 9). Carbamazepine is associated with a 1% risk of neural tube defects.[56-61] Concurrent folic acid 5 mg daily up to week 12 of pregnancy is recommended. Neural tube defects should be screened for by detailed ultrasound scan and alpha-fetoprotein (AFP) estimation at week 16 to 24.

Lithium

Lithium is used extensively to treat affective disorders. Exposure in pregnancy has been linked with Ebstein's anomaly, a cardiac abnormality in which the tricuspid valve is displaced into the right ventricle.[62,63] Initial data from an international register of lithium-exposed babies suggested that first-trimester exposure conferred a fivefold increase in the rate of congenital cardiovascular malformations and a 400-fold increase in the rate of Ebstein's anomaly. However, data from this register are subject to bias from over-reporting of abnormal outcomes. Several more recent cohort and case–control studies examined the effect of first trimester lithium exposure. In a recent prospective case–control study[64] involving 148 women who had taken lithium during part or all of the first trimester, no significant difference in the incidence of fetal malformation, spontaneous abortion, prematurity or stillbirth between the two groups was found.

Overall, available data on lithium exposure are consistent with an increased risk of cardiovascular abnormality, although the magnitude of the risk is probably much less than previously thought.[65]

Neonatal toxicity has also been reported with lithium.[66,67] A 'floppy baby' syndrome has been described with hypotonicity and cyanosis.[68] In women treated during the third trimester, the dose should be reduced by up to 50% just before delivery to minimise the risk of toxicity in mother and fetus. As the puerperium is a period of particular risk for bipolar women, lithium should not be stopped completely. A five-year follow-up study of 60 children exposed to lithium *in utero* found no evidence of abnormal development.[68]

Guidelines for lithium use during pregnancy

1   Lithium should only be used in women of child-bearing potential where there is a strong clinical need. Women must be advised that reliable contraception is essential.

2   Lithium should not be given during the first trimester unless absolutely necessary. The cardiovascular system is most vulnerable to teratogenic insult during days 20 to 45 after conception.

3   In women maintained on lithium it may be possible to gradually withdraw the medication before conception, but the rate of relapse is high if the medication is stopped abruptly.

4   A fetal echocardiogram at week 16 to 18 of pregnancy is recommended for women exposed during the first trimester. This can diagnose Ebstein's anomaly and other malformations.

5   When lithium is used, increasing doses will usually be necessary and frequent monitoring of plasma levels is required. Lithium should be given in small, divided doses to avoid peak levels that may be toxic to the fetus or neonate.

Sodium valproate

Sodium valproate is associated with teratogenic effects; in particular, the risk of neural tube defects is 1–2% (*see* Chapter 9).[69,70] There have also been reports of congenital cardiac defects, hypospadias, polydactyly and minor facial malformations, but it remains unclear whether these malformations are due to epilepsy itself.[71,72] Women taking sodium valproate should take folic acid 5 mg daily up to week 12 of pregnancy. Prenatal investigations to detect neural tube defects, including measurement of alpha-fetoprotein and amniocentesis, are recommended.

Antimanic agents and breastfeeding (Table 10.2)

About a third of the maternal daily dose of lithium passes into breast milk[75–77] and this level of exposure may lead to toxicity in the infant.[73–75] Mothers taking lithium should be advised against breastfeeding. If they choose to do so, the infant's plasma lithium levels should be closely monitored.

A breastfeeding infant will achieve plasma carbamazepine levels of about 25–60% of those in the mother, which are not considered significant.[76,77] The amount ingested by the baby is probably less than 10% of the therapeutic dose for an infant. Carbamazepine may be given during breastfeeding.

The infant may ingest up to 5% of the total maternal daily dose of sodium valproate[78,79] and breastfeeding appears to be safe.

Table 10.2: Safety of antimanic agents in pregnancy and lactation

Drug	Pregnancy	Breastfeeding
Valproate	Increased risk of neural tube defects (1–2%)	Safe
Lithium	Increased risk of cardiac malformations	Avoid significant amounts in breast milk
Carbamazepine	Increased risk of neural tube defects (0.5–1%)	Safe

Schizophrenia and related psychoses

There is controversy about whether psychotic illnesses tend to worsen or improve during pregnancy and also about whether babies born to schizophrenic mothers are at increased risk of congenital malformations even without drug exposure.

Acute psychosis is a medical and obstetric emergency. Psychosis may prevent women from obtaining proper prenatal care through denial of the pregnancy or delusions about the fetus. Women who first develop symptoms of psychotic illness in pregnancy require thorough evaluation to rule out organic causes for the change in mental status. Women maintained on antipsychotic medication should be advised to discuss a planned pregnancy with the doctor as soon as possible.

There are very few data on the effects of antipsychotic drugs in the treatment of psychoses in pregnancy; most information concerns their use for hyperemesis gravidarum.[80–83] In addition, many of the studies have flawed methodology and conflicting results. There is most documented experience with the phenothiazines and butyrophenones.

The use of depot antipsychotic preparations in pregnancy is not encouraged. There are no published data on the effects of zuclopenthixol, flupenthixol, pipothiazine and fluphenazine depot preparations in pregnancy. These agents cannot, if necessary, be withdrawn rapidly and the dose cannot be reduced towards delivery to limit neonatal withdrawal symptoms. Depot preparations should only be used where compliance is a problem.

Exposure to antipsychotics during the third trimester has been associated with neonatal toxicity. Symptoms include tremor, increased muscle tone, abnormal movements and feeding difficulties. Some experts suggest that drug therapy should be gradually withdrawn during the three to four weeks before delivery to minimise such effects. However, this is a difficult clinical decision because of the risk of relapse and discontinuing treatment may be inappropriate.

Phenothiazines

A recent meta-analysis of studies investigating pregnancy outcome following phenothiazine exposure concluded that there is a small, but statistically significant, increase in the overall risk of fetal abnormality. However, the authors also state that psychotic illness may confer the greatest increase in risk of poor fetal outcome.[6] There are not enough data to establish that one agent is safer than another. Most experience is with chlorpromazine and trifluoperazine.

Other neuroleptics

Two small studies found no association between the use of haloperidol for hyperemesis gravidarum and congenital malformations.[80–81]

There is insufficient information to recommend the use of sulpiride or pimozide. However, limited data from studies of sulpiride in vomiting in early pregnancy do not suggest that it has adverse fetal effects.[82,83]

Information on the effects of clozapine in pregnancy is limited to isolated case reports only.[84] These do not suggest that clozapine is a potent teratogen but its use in pregnancy is not recommended.

Newer antipsychotics

There is insufficient information regarding the effects of risperidone, olanzapine and sertindole in human pregnancy and their use is not recommended.

Antipsychotics and breastfeeding (Table 10.3)

Chlorpromazine concentrations in breast milk have been reported to be higher than in maternal plasma.[85] No information is available on the relationship between milk and plasma concentrations. Haloperidol is excreted into breast milk in small amounts.[86,87] It is suggested that mothers receiving antipsychotics may breastfeed, but babies should be observed for sedative effects. There is insufficient information on the safety of clozapine,[88] sulpiride, pimozide, risperidone and sertindole in breastfeeding.

Table 10.3: Safety of antipsychotics in pregnancy and lactation

Class	Drug	Pregnancy	Breastfeeding
Phenothiazines	Chlorpromazine Trifluoperazine	Probably safe: treatment of choice	Use with caution
	Fluphenazine	Limited outcome data – avoid	Avoid
Butyrophenones	Haloperidol	Probably safe Treatment of choice	Limited data – use with caution
	Droperidol	Limited outcome data – avoid	No data
Thioxanthenes	Flupenthixol Zuclopenthixol	Limited outcome data – avoid	Limited data – use with caution
Atypicals	Amisulpride Clozapine Sulpiride Olanzapine Quetiapine Risperidone Sertindole	Limited outcome data – avoid	Best avoided

Anxiety

Anxiety attacks may occur in pregnancy in response to concerns about the possible dangers involved. However, in some women anxiety impairs the ability to undertake simple, everyday tasks. Physical symptoms, such as gastrointestinal disturbances, tachycardia, tremor, sleep disturbance and poor concentration, may be present. Specific phobias are often managed by cognitive and behavioural therapies.

Non-drug treatments are preferred for anxiety states in pregnancy although pharmacological intervention may be required in severe cases.[89] Tricyclic antidepressants have been used to treat panic disorders, but there is more experience with the benzodiazepines (Table 10.4).

Table 10.4: Safety of antidepressants and benzodiazepines in pregnancy and lactation

Class	Drug	Pregnancy	Breastfeeding
Tricyclic and related drugs	Amitriptyline Imipramine	Probably safe	Probably safe
Benzodiazepines	Diazepam Chlordiazepoxide	Minimal risk	Short-term use probably safe Use short-acting agent Monitor infant for sedation
SSRIs	Fluoxetine	Probably safe May be used if other agents inappropriate	Use with caution (*see* Table 10.1)

The potential risk of oral clefts resulting from maternal ingestion of benzodiazepines has not been realised. Large case–control studies have shown no increased risk of cleft palate in those infants exposed to benzodiazepines *in utero*.[90] Frequent benzodiazepine ingestion is also associated with substantial alcohol consumption and other illicit drug use. This may have confounded some studies investigating the effects of benzodiazepine exposure *in utero*.

Benzodiazepines, particularly diazepam and chlordiazepoxide, have been associated with neonatal drug withdrawal.[29-31] Where possible, benzodiazepines should be stopped or the dose reduced before delivery.

Summary

- Non-pharmacological treatments, such as cognitive and behavioural therapies, should be considered where possible.
- Drugs with which there is most clinical experience during pregnancy are preferred.
- In general, women who become pregnant while taking a psychotropic agent should continue their medication unless it is thought that this can safely be reduced or stopped.
- The lowest effective dose of pyschotropic drugs should be used for the shortest possible period. Medication should be reviewed regularly.
- Where possible, psychoactive drugs should be withdrawn about three to four weeks before delivery to minimise the risk of neonatal withdrawal effects.

References

1　Kumar R and Robson K (1978) In *Mental Illness in Pregnancy and the Puerperium* (ed M Sandler). Oxford University Press, Oxford.
2　Cox JL (1979) Psychiatric morbidity and pregnancy. A controlled study of 263 semi-rural Ugandan women. *Br J Psychiat.* **309**: 1282–5.
3　Cox JL (1982) Prospective study of the psychiatric disorders of pregnancy. *Br J Psychiat.* **140**: 111–17.
4　Myers JK *et al.* (1984) Prospective study of the psychiatric disorders of pregnancy. *Arch Gen Psych.* **41**: 959–67.
5　Kuller JA, Katz VL, McMahon MJ *et al.* (1996) Pharmacological treatment of psychiatric disease in pregnancy and lactation: fetal and neonatal effects. *Obstet Gynecol.* **87**: 789–94.
6　Altshuler LL and Szuba M (1994) Course of psychiatric disorders in pregnancy. *Neurol Clin.* **12**: 613–35.
7　McElhatton PR *et al.* (1996) The outcome of pregnancy in 689 women exposed to therapeutic doses of antidepressants. A collaborative study of the European Network of Teratology Information Services (ENTIS). *Reprod Toxicol.* **10**: 285–94.

8   Goldberg HL and Szuba MP (1994) Psychotropic drugs in pregnancy and lactation. *Int J Psychiat Med.* **24**: 129–49.

9   Crombie DL *et al.* (1975) Fetal effects of tranquilisers in pregnancy. *N Engl J Med.* **293**: 198–9.

10 Kuenssberg EV and Knox JD (1972) Imipramine in pregnancy. *BMJ.* **2**: 292.

11 Eggermont E (1973) Withdrawal symptoms in neonates associated with maternal imipramine therapy. *Lancet.* **2**: 680.

12 Bromiker R *et al.* (1994) Apparent intrauterine fetal withdrawal from clomipramine hydrochloride. *JAMA.* **272**: 1722–3.

13 Webster PA (1973) Withdrawal symptoms in neonates associated with maternal antidepressant therapy. *Lancet.* **2**: 318–9.

14 Ben Musa A *et al.* (1979) Neonatal effects of maternal clomipramine therapy. *Arch Dis Child.* **54**: 405.

15 Eggermont E (1980) Neonatal effects of maternal therapy with tricylcic antidepressant drugs. *Arch Dis Child.* **55**: 81.

16 Idanpaan-Heikkila J and Saxen L (1973) Possible teratogenicity of imipramine/chloropyramine. *Lancet.* **2**: 282–4.

17 Dahl ML *et al.* (1997) Paroxetine withdrawal syndrome in a neonate. *Br J Psychiat.* **171**: 391–4.

18 Chambers C D *et al.* (1996) Birth outcomes in pregnant women taking fluoxetine. *N Engl J Med.* **335**: 1010–15.

19 Spencer MJ (1993) Fluoxetine hydrochloride toxicity in a neonate. *Pediatrics.* **92**: 721–2.

20 Kent LSW and Laidlaw JDD (1995) Suspected congenital sertraline dependance. *Br J Psychiat.* **167**: 412–13.

21 O'Connor M *et al.* (1981) Intrauterine effects of phenothiazines. *Med J Aust.* **1**: 416–17.

22 Tamer A *et al.* (1969) Phenothiazine-induced extrapyramidal dysfunction in the neonate. *J Pediatr.* **75**: 479–80.

23 Prenner BM (1977) Neonatal withdrawal syndrome associated with hydroxyzine hydrochloride. *Am J Dis Child.* **131**: 529–30.

24 Zelson C *et al.* (1973) Neonatal narcotic addiction. *N Engl J Med.* **289**: 1216–20.

25 Zelson C *et al.* (1971) Neonatal narcotic addiction: a 10-year observation. *Pediatrics.* **48**: 178–89.

26 Blatman S (1974) Narcotic poisoning of children: (1) through accidental ingestion of methadone and (2) *in utero. Pediatr Clin.* **54**: 329–32.

27 Tenenbein M *et al.* (1996) Neonatal withdrawal from maternal volatile substance abuse. *Arch Dis Child.* **74**: F204–F207.

28 Hanson J W *et al.* (1976) Fetal alcohol syndrome. *JAMA.* **235**: 1458–60.

29 Bergman U *et al.* (1992) Effects of exposure to benzodiazepine during fetal life. *Lancet.* **340**: 694–6.

30 Rementeria JL and Bhatt K (1977) Withdrawal symptoms in neonates from intrauterine exposure to diazepam. *J Pediatr.* **90**: 123–6.

31 Athinarayanan P *et al.* (1976) Chlordiazepoxide withdrawal in the neonate. *Am J Obstet Gynecol.* **124**: 212–13.

32 Schardein JL (1993) *Chemically Induced Birth Defects* (2nd edn), pp. 219–21. Marcel Dekker, New York.

33 Goldstein DJ and Marvel DE (1993) Psychotropic medications during pregnancy: risk to fetus. *JAMA.* **270**: 2177.

34 Chambers CD *et al.* (1996) Birth outcomes in pregnant women taking fluoxetine. *N Engl J Med.* **335**: 1010–15.

35 Robert E (1996) Treating depression in pregnancy. *N Engl J Med.* **335**(14): 1056–8.

36 Rosa FW (1994) Medicaid antidepressant pregnancy exposure outcomes. *Reprod Toxicol.* **8**: 444.

37 Repke JT and Berger NG (1984) Electroconvulsive therapy in pregnancy. *Obstet Gynecol.* **63**: S39–S41.

38 Sobel DE (1960) Fetal damage due to ECT, insulin coma, chlorpromazine or reserpine. *Arch Gen Psych.* **2**: 606–11.

39 Goldstein HH *et al.* (1941) Shock therapy in psychosis complicating pregnancy, a case report. *Am J Psychiatr.* **98**: 201–2.

40 Impastato DJ *et al.* (1964) Electric and insulin shock therapy during pregnancy. *Dis Nerv Syst.* **25**: 542–6.

41 Remick RA and Maurice WL (1978) ECT in pregnancy. *Am J Psychiatr.* **135**: 761–2.

42 Forssman H (1955) Follow-up study of 16 children whose mothers were given electric convulsive therapy during gestation. *Acta Psychiatr Neurol Scand.* **30**: 437–41.

43 Miller LJ (1994) Clinical strategies for the use of psychotropic drugs during pregnancy. *Hosp Comm Psychiat.* **45**: 444–50.

44 Ferrill MJ *et al.* (1992) ECT during pregnancy and pharmacologic consideration. *Convuls Ther.* **8**: 186–200.

45 Misri S and Sivertz K (1991) Tricyclic drugs in pregnancy and lactation: a preliminary report. *Int J Psych Med.* **21**: 157–71.

46 Bader TF and Newman K (1980) Amitriptyline in human breast milk and the nursing infant's serum. *Am J Psychiat.* **137**: 855–64.

47 Brixen-Rasmussen L (1982) Amitriptyline and nortriptyline excretion in human breast milk. *Psychopharmacology.* **72**: 94–5.

48 Wisner KL and Perel JM (1991) Serum nortriptyline levels in nursing mothers and their infants. *Am J Psychiat.* **148**: 1234–6.

49 Stancer HC and Reed KL (1986) Desipramine and 2-hydroxydesipramine in human breast milk and the nursing infant's serum. *Am J Psychiat.* **143**: 1597–600.

50 O'Brien TE (1974) Excretion of drugs in human breast milk. *Am J Hosp Pharm.* **31**: 844–54.

51 Pons G *et al.* (1990) Moclobemide in human breast milk. *Br J Clin Pharm.* **30**: 267–71.

52 Hale T (1999) *Medications and Mothers' Milk 1998–1999* (7th edn). Pharmasoft Medical Publishing, Texas.

53 Lester BM, Cucca J, Andreozzi L *et al.* (1993) Possible association between fluoxetine hydrochloride and colic in an infant. *J Am Acad Child Adolesc Psychiatry.* **32**(6): 1253–5.

54 Targum SD and Gershon ES (1981) *Pregnancy: maternal effects and fetal outcome* (eds Schulman and Simpson). Academic Press, New York.

55 de Swiet M (1995) *Medical Disorders in Obstetric Practice* (3rd edn). Blackwell Scientific, Oxford.

56 Dalessio DJ (1985) Seizure disorders and pregnancy. *N Engl J Med.* **312**: 559–63.

57 Holmes LB *et al.* (1990) Teratogenic effects of anticonvulsants. *Teratology.* **41**: 565.

58 Jones KL *et al.* (1989) Pattern of malformations in the children of women treated with carbamazepine during pregnancy. *N Engl J Med.* **320**: 1661–6.

59   Nakane Y *et al.* (1980) Multi-institutional study on the teratogenicity and fetal toxicity of anti-epileptic drugs: a report of a collabrative study group in Japan. *Epilepsia.* **21**: 663–80.

60   Paulson GW and Paulson RB (1981) Teratogenic effects of anticonvulsants. *Arch Neurol.* **40**: 140–1.

61   Rosa FW (1991) Spina bifida in infants of women taking carbamazepine. *N Engl J Med.* **324**: 674–7.

62   Zalstein E *et al.* (1990) A case–control study on the association between first-trimester exposure to lithium and Ebstein's anomaly. *Am J Cardiol.* **65**: 817–88.

63   Nora JJ *et al.* (1974) Lithium, Ebstein's anomaly and other congenital heart defects. *Lancet.* **2**: 594.

64   Jacobson SJ (1992) Prospective multicentre study of pregnancy outcome after lithium exposure in first trimester. *Lancet.* **339**: 530–3.

65   Cohen LS *et al.* (1994) A re-evaluatiion of risk of *in utero* exposure to lithium. *JAMA.* **271**: 146–50.

66   Rane A *et al.* (1978) Effects of maternal lithium therapy in a newborn infant. *J Pediatr.* **93**: 296–7.

67   Schou M (1975) Lithium and placenta. *Am J Obstet Gynecol.* **122**: 541.

68   Woody JN *et al.* (1971) Lithium toxicity in a newborn. *Pediatrics.* **47**: 94–6.

69   Center for Disease Control, US and Department of Health and Human Services (1983) Valproate: a new cause of birth defects – report from Italy and follow-up from France. *MMWR.* **32**: 438–9.

70   Lammer EJ *et al.* (1987) Teratogen update: valproic acid. *Teratology.* 35: 465–73.

71   Koch S *et al.* (1983) Major malformations in children of epileptic parents – due to epilepsy or its treatment? *J Pediatr.* **103**: 1007–8.

72   DiLerberti JD *et al.* (1984) The fetal valproate syndrome. *Am J Med Genet.* **25**: 32–8.

73   Sykes PA *et al.* (1976) Lithium carbonate and breastfeeding. *BMJ.* **4**: 1299.

74   Shimizu M *et al.* (1981) A few findings on lithium levels in mothers' milk. *Seishin Shinkeigaku Zasshi.* **83**: 399–405.

75   Skausig OB and Schou M (1977) Breast feeding during lithium treatment. *Ugeskr Laeger.* **39**: 400–1.

76   Kaneko S *et al.* (1979) The levels of anticonvulsants in breast milk. *Br J Clin Pharm.* **7**: 624.

77   Niebyl JR *et al.* (1979) Carbamazepine levels in pregnancy and lactation. *Obstet Gynecol.* **53**: 139.

78   Nau H *et al.* (1981) Valproic acid and its metabolites: placental transfer, neonatal pharmacokinetics, transfer via the mother's milk and clinical status in neonates of epileptic mothers. *J Pharm Exp Ther.* **219**: 768–77.

79   Rimmer EM and Richens A (1985) An update on sodium valproate. *Pharmacotherapy.* **5**: 171–84.

80   Hanson GW and Oakley GP (1975) Haloperidol and limb deformities. *JAMA.* **231**: 26.

81   Kullander S and Kallen B (1976) A prospective study of drugs and pregnancy. *Acta Obstet Gynecol Scand.* **55**: 25–33.

82   Crepin G *et al.* (1977) Sulpiride treatment of hyperemesis gravidarum. *Rev Franc Gynecol.* **72**(7–9): 539–46.

83   Goni JA (1972) Treatment of the vomiting syndrome in pregnancy with sulpiride. *Sem Med.* **140**(10): 296–8.

84 Walderman MD and Safferman AZ (1993) Pregnancy and clozapine. *Am J Psychiat.* **150**: 168–9.

85 Wiles DH *et al.* (1978) Chlorpromazine levels in plasma and milk of nursing mothers. *Br J Clin Pharm.* **5**: 273.

86 Whalley LJ *et al.* (1981) Haloperidol secreted in breast milk. *BMJ.* **282**: 1746–7.

87 Stewart RB *et al.* (1980) Haloperidol excretion in human milk. *Am J Psychiat.* **137**: 849.

88 Barnas C *et al.* (1994) Clozapine concentrations in maternal and fetal plasma, amniotic fluid and breast milk. *Am J Psychiat.* **151**: 945.

89 McGrath C, Buist A and Norman TR (1999) Treatment of anxiety during pregnancy. Effects of drug treatment on the developing fetus. *Drug Safety.* **20**(2): 171–86.

90 Rosenberg L *et al.* (1983) Lack of relation of oral clefts to diazepam use during pregnancy. *N Engl J Med.* **309**: 1282–3.

CHAPTER ELEVEN

Infections

David Finnigan

Introduction

Infections commonly complicate pregnancy. Although many are minor, self-limiting illnesses, some may cause harm to the mother, the fetus or both. TORCH, an acronym for toxoplasmosis, rubella, cytomegalovirus (CMV) and herpes, was first used in 1971 to highlight those infections that can cause congenital disease. This term is no longer recommended as it omits other infections that can harm the fetus, including syphilis, parvovirus B19, listeria, human immunodeficiency virus (HIV), and hepatitis B.[1] This chapter gives an overview of some of the infections that may occur during pregnancy and the therapeutic issues raised by these in the context of UK practice. Breastfeeding is discussed where relevant. At the end of the chapter, Table 11.2 outlines a summary of the main points.

Viral infections

Rubella

Rubella (German measles) is caused by an RNA virus. It has an incubation period of 14–21 days and is infective from about one week before, until four days after, the appearance of any rash. It is usually a mild childhood infection, characterised by a generalised rash that may be preceded by upper respiratory symptoms and posterior cervical lymphadenopathy. In adults, a transient arthralgia may occur as the rash begins to fade. Frequently there is no rash.[2] In the UK, the incidence of rubella in pregnancy is very low, as most women are immune. Thirty-two cases of rubella occurring during pregnancy were reported in England and Wales in 1996, and only three cases in 1997.[3] The high maternal immunity rates are largely due to the selective immunisation programme for schoolgirls and women introduced in 1970.[4] In 1988, MMR vaccination for all children at 13 months was introduced, and since 1996 an additional dose of MMR has been given with the diphtheria, tetanus and polio pre-school booster.

Although rubella is a mild illness for the mother the effect on the fetus can be catastrophic, resulting in miscarriage, stillbirth, intrauterine growth retardation or severe malformations. Live-born infected infants most commonly present with cardiac defects, neurological abnormalities (microcephaly, cerebral palsy, mental handicap), ocular defects (cataract, microphthalmia, retinitis), deafness, hepatosplenomegaly, jaundice and purpura. Even in those not clinically affected at birth, virus may persist in the lens of the eye and the middle ear, leading to progressive cataract and deafness. The risk of major fetal malformations is highest if infection occurs during the first trimester, approaching 100% for infection occurring within the first 11 weeks of gestation. After 17 weeks gestation the risk is negligible.[5] The risk of fetal infection is probably negligible with periconceptional maternal rubella, with no reported cases of fetal infection when the mother's rash appears before, or within 11 days after, the last menstrual period.[6]

Identification of rubella infection during pregnancy can be difficult. Many viruses can cause a similar rash to rubella and asymptomatic infection commonly occurs. In one study, in 25% of cases of congenital rubella there was no maternal history of illness, rash, or contact with rubella. In 15% of cases there was a history of maternal contact with rubella but without any apparent illness afterwards.[7,8]

If rubella is suspected, or if maternal exposure to rubella occurs, serology should be checked as soon as possible. Prior history of rubella, previous immunisation, or immunity demonstrated on antenatal testing is no excuse for not investigating as reinfection can occur, although the risk of fetal abnormality is much less in this situation.[9] High titres of rubella-specific IgG within the incubation period of 14–21 days suggest previous infection and immunity. Seroconversion or a significant rise in titre is diagnostic of infection. The presence of specific IgM is highly suggestive of recent infection, although IgM can persist for several months and its presence may be due to infection that occurred prior to the pregnancy.[10] Early diagnosis is essential, as possible termination of the pregnancy should be discussed with the pregnant woman if first-trimester infection occurs.

Prenatal diagnosis of congenital rubella is possible but is not standard practice. It requires cordocentesis and detection of specific IgM in fetal blood, or isolation of the virus following amniocentesis or chorionic villus sampling.[8,10] The presence of specific IgM or persistence of specific IgG In the infant confirms congenital infection.

It is routine antenatal practice to check the rubella status of all pregnant women. If a woman is non-immune she should be advised to avoid contact with cases of suspected rubella and to report any rashes. Post-partum vaccination should also be offered. Rubella immunisation is with a live attenuated vaccine; it should not be given during pregnancy and pregnancy avoided for one month following vaccination. There have been no reports, however, of fetal abnormality following inadvertent immunisation of pregnant women.[2,4]

Breastfeeding is not contraindicated in mothers with rubella infection or following rubella vaccination.[11]

Cytomegalovirus (CMV)

Cytomegalovirus (CMV) is a member of the herpes virus family. It lies dormant after acute infection and may reactivate at times of stress or impaired immunity. Infection can occur following close or sexual contact, blood transfusion, organ transplantation or transplacental transmission.[12] Exposure is common by adult life, with seropositivity ranging from 40–80%.[12] Infection is usually subclinical or causes a mild, glandular fever-like illness.[12] Infection can be severe, however, if immunity is impaired, in neonates, and in a small number of healthy individuals. Complications include hepatitis, pneumonitis, retinitis, encephalitis, and Guillain–Barré syndrome. Recurrent infection is less severe but is more common. CMV is the most common cause of congenital viral infection.[13]

Primary infection occurs in 1–4% of all pregnancies with a 30–40% risk of transmission to the fetus, although only 10% of infected infants will be symptomatic at birth.[12,14] The risk of transmission with recurrent maternal infection is less than 1% and these infants are even less likely to be born with symptomatic disease.[12] It is estimated that the incidence of congenital CMV ranges from 0.5–2% of all live births.[12,14]

Congenital infection is associated with intrauterine growth retardation and may cause miscarriage or stillbirth.[12] Infants born with symptomatic disease present with a variety of problems, most frequently hepatosplenomegaly, jaundice, petechiae, microcephaly, and periventricular calcification.[13,15] Less commonly, chorioretinitis, optic atrophy, deafness and pneumonitis can occur. Infants presenting with abnormal neurological signs have a worse prognosis than those who do not, with severe handicap at follow-up in 70% and 30% respectively.[15] The outlook is much better if the infant is asymptomatic at birth, although 5–15% of such infants will develop problems, especially hearing loss.[13,14]

Infection occurring during pregnancy is usually not suspected, as most women are asymptomatic. Seroconversion or a significant rise in CMV-specific IgG titres confirms the diagnosis. The presence of specific IgM is suggestive of primary infection, although IgM can persist for several months and 10% of women with recurrent infection have IgM antibodies.[14] Even if there is evidence of previous infection this does not exclude the possibility of fetal infection from recurrent maternal infection.

Prenatal diagnosis of fetal infection is difficult. Detection of specific IgM in fetal blood, obtained by cordocentesis, is probably diagnostic, although there is a high false negative rate. IgM is not detectable in the first half of pregnancy, probably because of immaturity of the fetal immune system.[13,14] Ultrasound abnormalities are usually a late finding and are not specific enough to make the diagnosis of congenital CMV infection. Currently the best way of making a diagnosis is by isolating the virus from amniotic fluid.[8] A positive diagnosis, however, does not predict the severity of congenital CMV infection and many infected infants will be asymptomatic.[14]

In the newborn infant a diagnosis of congenital CMV infection is usually made from viral cultures of urine or saliva within the first three weeks of life.[8,12] Detection of specific IgM within the first three weeks of birth is also diagnostic.[8]

There is no effective therapy for CMV infection in pregnancy.[14] There is currently work on developing a safe and effective vaccine.[12] Antenatal screening is not routinely carried out due to the limitations of the currently available tests, as discussed previously. Pregnant women should be reassured that even with primary infection the risk of fetal injury is low.

Breastfeeding is not contraindicated if a mother is diagnosed as having either primary or recurrent CMV infection, although CMV may be excreted into breast milk. There is concern, however, that very premature babies may acquire symptomatic CMV infection via breast milk. It is probably wise in such infants to avoid breastfeeding or to treat expressed breast milk to inactivate the virus.[16]

Chickenpox (*Varicella zoster*)

Chickenpox is caused by primary infection with *Varicella zoster*, a DNA herpes virus. It has an incubation period of 10–20 days and is infective from 48 hours before the appearance of the rash until all the vesicles crust over, which takes about 6 days.[17] It is a common childhood illness and most adults are immune, with only 10% of pregnant women susceptible.[18–20] Chickenpox is usually more severe in adults, with an increased risk of complications such as varicella pneumonitis. Although it is uncertain whether chickenpox is likely to be even more severe in pregnancy, the risk of pneumonitis appears to be particularly high in the latter half of pregnancy.[20]

Chickenpox is reported to occur in one per 2000 pregnancies, although this is probably an underestimate.[18,20] There is a 2% risk of fetal abnormality with infection occurring in the first half of pregnancy.[21] The most common abnormalities are dermatomal skin scarring, eye defects (microphthalmia, chorioretinitis, cataracts), limb hypoplasia and neurological abnormalities (microcephaly, mental handicap, bowel and bladder sphincter dysfunction).[17,19] Congenital abnormalities have not been reported following maternal chickenpox after 20 weeks gestation.[21] The danger to the fetus later on in pregnancy is from symptomatic varicella infection, which becomes increasingly likely as gestation progresses. If maternal chickenpox occurs one to four weeks before delivery, a third of newborn infants develop clinical varicella infection despite the protection of passively acquired maternal antibody.[21] Infection is particularly severe if maternal chickenpox occurs four days before delivery and up to two days post-partum, due to the lack of maternal antibody. Without treatment, up to 20–30% of these infants will die, usually from severe pneumonia or fulminant hepatitis.[17–19]

There is a lack of evidence on how best to manage chickenpox in pregnancy and specialist advice should be obtained in all cases. Box 11.1 outlines the recommendations of the Royal College of Obstetricians and Gynaecologists, UK.[19] This broadly agrees with the recommendations of a recent review prepared for the UK Advisory Group on Chickenpox.[20,22] *Varicella zoster* immunoglobulin (VZIG) is available from the Public Health Laboratory Service (PHLS), although supplies are limited. At present PHLS is only issuing VZIG for antibody negative pregnant women who present with a history of contact within the first 20 weeks gestation or within three weeks of expected delivery.[23] When supplies permit, however, PHLS issues VZIG for all antibody negative pregnant contacts (personal communication, PHLS).

A live, attenuated vaccine is currently only available on a named patient basis from SmithKline Beecham or Pasteur Mérieux. If this was to become more freely available, there is debate about whether this should be offered as part of a universal or selective immunisation programme. Selective immunisation would require testing all women of child-bearing age without a history of chickenpox. Of these, only 15% will be found to be non-immune and require vaccination.[18,20] Post-partum vaccination could be offered to those susceptible women already pregnant.

Breastfeeding is not contraindicated in mothers with chickenpox, although if lesions are present around the nipple it is best avoided until the lesions crust over.[11]

Box 11.1: Recommendations on management of chickenpox in pregnancy*

Suspected varicella contact

1 Assess degree of likely exposure.
2 If previous history of chickenpox then assume immune.
3 If uncertain or no past history of chickenpox, check serology (up to 85% will be immune).
4 If not immune and less than 20 weeks gestation, give *Varicella zoster* immunoglobulin (VZIG).
5 If greater than 20 weeks gestation, there is no risk of congenital varicella infection but there is a risk of maternal pneumonitis.
6 If chickenpox develops or there is serological evidence of infection (specific IgM or rising titre of IgG) within the first 20 weeks gestation, there is a 2% risk of congenital varicella infection and the woman should be counselled regarding this.
7 Detailed ultrasound scan at 16–20 weeks gestation or five weeks after infection, whichever is sooner, should be considered.
8 Neonatal eye examination should be organised.

Presents with chickenpox

1 Isolate from all other pregnant women and neonates.
2 If in the second half of pregnancy and less than 24 hours after the development of the rash, treatment with oral aciclovir should be considered to try and reduce the severity and duration of the illness.
3 Varicella pneumonia requires treatment with IV aciclovir.
4 If practical, delivery should be delayed until 5–7 days after the onset of maternal illness to allow passive transfer of antibodies.
5 If delivery occurs within five days of maternal infection, or if the mother develops chickenpox within two days of giving birth, the neonate should be given VZIG as soon as possible.
6 If neonatal infection occurs then this should be treated with aciclovir.

* Royal College of Obstetricians and Gynaecologists, UK guidelines 1997.

Human parvovirus

Parvovirus B19 is a DNA virus that was first discovered in 1975 and is the cause of erythema infectiosum, also known as fifth disease or slapped cheek syndrome. It is also the main cause of aplastic crisis in patients with haemolytic anaemias. It has an incubation period of 4–14 days, but this can be as long as 20 days; infectivity is up until the appearance of the rash.[24] Seroprevalence is about 60% in adults.[24] It is usually a mild infection of children, characterised by a raised, fiery red rash on the cheeks and followed by a mild, macular rash mainly on the limbs and trunk. Joint pains can occur, more often in adults. Many cases are asymptomatic.

The first case of congenital infection was reported in 1984. The chance of a pregnant woman becoming infected is small, as most are immune. If a woman is susceptible then the risk of infection following exposure is about 16%; however, if the exposure is to an infected child living in the same household this risk increases to 30%.[25] If a pregnant woman is infected, the risk of transmitting the virus to the fetus is approximately 20%.[26] Infection can result in spontaneous abortion, stillbirth, or fetal anaemia and hydrops fetalis.[24,26,27] The excess risk of fetal death is confined to the first 20 weeks of gestation and is estimated to be about 9%.[26] There is no convincing evidence that infection results in congenital abnormalities.[2,26,28,29]

In most cases maternal parvovirus infection will not be suspected, although many patients will have polyarthralgia, fever, and non-specific rash.[25] If infection is suspected, then demonstrating seroconversion will confirm the diagnosis.[1,30] The presence of specific IgM is also suggestive, although IgM can persist for several months. The virus cannot be cultured but DNA amplification tests have been used to identify the virus in maternal blood, amniotic fluid and fetal blood.[8]

It is uncertain how best to manage parvovirus infection during pregnancy. Sequential ultrasound may be useful in detecting the development of hydrops fetalis.[31,32] Fetal blood samples obtained by cordocentesis can indicate the severity of the aplastic crisis; *in utero* transfusions or early delivery and transfusions may be beneficial, although it is thought that up to a third of cases of hydrops resolve spontaneously.[30–32] Therapeutic abortion is inappropriate as intrauterine infection is embryocidal, not teratogenic.

If a pregnant woman is diagnosed as being infected she should be reassured that the most likely outcome is a healthy term infant.

Hepatitis B

Hepatitis B is caused by hepatitis B virus (HBV), which primarily infects liver cells. Transmission most commonly occurs following sexual contact, blood-to-blood contact or perinatally from mother to child. The incubation period is between 2–6 months. Symptomatic cases present with jaundice, but it is estimated that 60–80% of acute infections are asymptomatic or only associated with mild, flu-like symptoms.[1,30] Ninety per cent of acute HBV infections resolve completely within six months. In the remainder a chronic carrier state develops, with persistence of hepatitis B surface antigen (HBsAg).[1] The prevalence of HBsAg in pregnant women is 0.1–0.2% in the UK.[33]

Infants of women infected with HBV are at high risk of acquiring hepatitis B, usually at the time of delivery.[33,34] Infectivity is particularly high if hepatitis B 'e' antigen (HBeAg) is present and low if antibody to

HBeAg (anti-HBe) is present. The risk of fetal transmission is 15–20% if the mother is HBsAg positive, 10% if she is anti-HBe positive and 70–90% if she is HBeAg positive.[1,33] Most neonatal infections result in asymptomatic carrier states, with a significant risk of cirrhosis and hepatocellular carcinoma later on in life.[33,34]

A carrier state can be prevented in over 90% of infants born to HBsAg or HBeAg positive mothers by giving passive immunisation with hepatitis B immunoglobulin (HBIG) combined with active immunisation with hepatitis B vaccine.[1,33,35] Current recommendation is to give this to infants born to mothers who are HBeAg positive, who are HBsAg positive without 'e' markers, or who have had acute hepatitis during pregnancy.[23] HBIG is given after birth, followed by a full course of hepatitis B vaccine. The first dose of vaccine is given soon after birth, followed by a further dose one month later and then a final dose six months after the first. Infants born to mothers who are HBsAg positive and who also have anti-HBe are given the course of vaccine but do not require HBIG.[23]

The Department of Health recommends screening all pregnant women for hepatitis B infection.[23] In 1995, most health authorities in England and Wales had a selective policy, screening pregnant women considered at risk of hepatitis B.[33] This policy has been shown to miss over 40% of HBsAg positive women.[33]

Breastfeeding is not contraindicated in mothers with chronic hepatitis B.[11]

HIV infection

Human immunodeficiency virus (HIV), a retrovirus, was first identified as the cause of acquired immunodeficiency syndrome (AIDS) in 1983. Prevalence varies with geography and is especially high in London where, on average one in 500 births are to HIV-infected mothers, compared to an overall rate of one in 6000 births for other parts of England and Wales.[36] In Scotland, prevalence is particularly high in Dundee and Edinburgh.[1] Mother-to-child transmission is the main cause of childhood infection, accounting for 85% of cases in the UK.[37] Transmission can occur before and during birth, or from breastfeeding which doubles the rate of transmission. A non-breastfeeding, untreated mother has a 15–20% risk of infecting her child.[38] It is estimated that about 300 infants are born to HIV-infected mothers each year in the UK, with over 75% of mothers undiagnosed at the time of birth.[37] Women often only discover they are infected when their child develops AIDS. About 20% of HIV-infected children develop AIDS or die in the first year of life, and most children will eventually develop AIDS.[37]

In 1994, it was shown that treating HIV-infected pregnant women with zidovudine reduces the risk of transmission to the child by about two-thirds.[38,39]

Zidovudine is now licensed for use in pregnancy and experience to date has shown no evidence of adverse effects on the fetus.[37] There is some evidence that Caesarean section may decrease the risk of mother-to-child transmission of HIV.[38] This is not advised as a preventative strategy until more data is available.

Identification of maternal HIV infection also directly benefits the mother. Advances in the treatment of HIV, especially with combination therapies, have improved survival.[38,40]

Although voluntary confidential antenatal testing has been available for some time, women have often not been offered testing even in areas of high HIV prevalence.[41] Many countries now routinely offer antenatal testing, with treatment of identified cases and avoidance of breastfeeding, which has led to a reduction in the number of infected children. This is in contrast to the UK where numbers are continuing to climb.[37] Following the recent recommendations of a working party set up to look at ways of reducing mother to baby transmission of HIV, all women are now to be offered HIV testing as an addition to routine antenatal screening tests.[37,42] This was to be fully implemented by December 2000 with a target that by December 2002 the uptake of antenatal HIV testing will be 90% or more.

If maternal HIV infection is diagnosed then support and counselling is vital, with involvement of specialist HIV services to advise on the treatment of both mother and child. A detailed review of treatment is beyond the scope of this book. Women should be informed that treatment during pregnancy and avoidance of breastfeeding greatly reduces the risk of transmission to the child, although the risk is still about 5%.

Bacterial and other infections

Respiratory infections

Upper respiratory tract infections are usually minor, self-limiting disorders that only require symptomatic relief. They include coryza (common cold), acute sinusitis, otitis media, and tonsillitis. Paracetamol is safe in pregnancy and is the preferred analgesic. Treatments containing a mixture of other ingredients, such as antihistamines, sympathomimetics or caffeine, are best avoided. Antibiotics are usually not required, but if used choice should be restricted to those known to be safe in pregnancy. Amoxycillin, erythromycin and cephalosporins are suitable choices and should be used in full adult doses.[43] Tetracyclines are contraindicated in pregnancy due to deposition in growing bones and teeth with resultant risk of fetal abnormalities.[44] Ciprofloxacin and other quinolones should be avoided because of adverse effects on developing cartilage in animal studies, although there is no evidence of teratogenicity in humans.[44]

Bacterial pneumonia is rare but can cause maternal death.[43] It is most commonly caused by *Streptococcus pneumoniae*, followed by *Haemophilus influenzae* and *Mycoplasma pneumoniae*.[45] Rarer infections are *Legionella pneumoniae* and *Listeria monocytogenes*. Hospital admission is required for monitoring and antibiotic therapy. Penicillin is the preferred treatment for pneumococcal pneumonia, or erythromycin if penicillin-allergic. Amoxycillin is the preferred treatment for haemophilus, unless culture results show resistance. Although tetracyclines are the preferred treatment for mycoplasma infection, these are contraindicated in pregnancy; therefore the best choice is erythromycin.

Breastfeeding can continue with the use of amoxycillin, erythromycin or a cephalosporin. Penicillins can theoretically cause sensitisation; therefore breastfeeding mothers should be advised to watch out for rashes or other signs of allergy in their infant. Tetracyclines are advised against, although they are probably safe to use as calcium inhibits absorption of the small amounts of tetracycline that pass into breast milk.[46,47]

Asymptomatic bacteriuria and urinary tract infection

Asymptomatic bacteriuria

Asymptomatic bacteriuria is defined as urinary tract infection in the absence of any symptoms, with greater than 100 000 bacteria/mL in a midstream urine sample.[48] It occurs in 5–10% of pregnancies, with similar prevalence in non-pregnant women.[48] *Escherichia coli* is the most common pathogen; other organisms include *Klebsiella* species, *Proteus* species, enterococci, staphylococci and group B streptococcus.[49,50] In non-pregnancy, asymptomatic bacteriuria is harmless and does not require treatment. In pregnancy, however, 20–30% of women will develop acute pyelonephritis unless treated.[48] Asymptomatic bacteriuria is also associated with an increased risk of premature birth.[2,48]

Treatment of asymptomatic bacteriuria reduces the risk of acute pyelonephritis by 75% and possibly reduces the risk of premature birth by about 40%.[48] It is uncertain how long a course of treatment should last. Single-dose therapy is not advised, but treatment for longer than three to seven days offers no additional advantage.[48,51] Amoxycillin, nitrofurantoin and cefalexin are safe to use in pregnancy (Table 11.1).[50,52,53] Amoxycillin is becoming less useful due to increasing rates of resistant *E. coli*.[50] Nitrofurantoin is contraindicated in women suspected or known to have glucose-6-phosphate dehydrogenase (G6PD) deficiency, due to the risk of haemolysis. Trimethoprim has not been shown to harm the fetus if given during pregnancy. It is not recommended, however, especially in the first trimester, as it is a folate antagonist and theoretically teratogenic.[44] Quinolones are not recommended because of adverse effects on developing cartilage in animal studies.[44] Co-amoxiclav (a beta-lactam/beta-lactamase inhibitor combination) is probably safe, but experience is limited.[53]

Antenatal screening for asymptomatic bacteriuria is standard practice in the UK. Urine cultures every four to six weeks until delivery are advised following treatment of an episode of bacteriuria.[50] More than three episodes of infection are an indication for prophylactic therapy with low-dose nitrofurantoin or cephalexin until delivery.[50]

Table 11.1: Treatment of asymptomatic bacteriuria or cystitis in pregnancy (all for seven days although three days is probably adequate)

Amoxycillin	500 mg three times daily
Cefalexin	500 mg three times daily
Nitrofurantoin	50 mg four times daily

Symptomatic urinary tract infection

Acute cystitis and acute pyelonephritis occur in 1–2% of pregnant women.[49] The treatment of cystitis is the same as that for asymptomatic bacteriuria (Table 11.1). Acute pyelonephritis in pregnancy requires hospitalisation. Intravenous broad-spectrum antibiotics are usually started while waiting for the results of urine and blood cultures. Reasonable choices are a third generation cephalosporin or a beta-lactam/beta-lactamase inhibitor combination (e.g. co-amoxiclav), with or without gentamicin, depending on how ill the patient is.[53] Gentamicin serum levels must be monitored carefully as there is a risk of toxicity to both mother and fetus.[49,53] When the patient is stable, oral treatment is started and continued for a further 10–14 days.

Urinary tract infection may recur in up to 60% of pregnant women following treatment of an episode of acute pyelonephritis.[49] Low-dose antibiotic prophylaxis may be considered, particularly if there is evidence of underlying renal disease.[44,49]

Breastfeeding can continue with the use of any of these recommended antibiotics. However, nitrofurantoin should be avoided if there is a possibility that the infant has G6PD deficiency.[47] Trimethoprim is safe to use.[46,47]

Listeriosis

Listeria monocytogenes, a Gram-positive bacillus, is an uncommon but serious cause of infection in pregnancy. In 1996, listeriosis was reported in 16 pregnancies in England and Wales.[54] Possible sources of infection are pâtés, unpasteurised milk, raw vegetables and soft cheeses (Brie, Camembert, blue-vein types). Several outbreaks in the past have been associated with contaminated prepared foods, although infections are usually sporadic.[1,55]

An infected pregnant woman may be asymptomatic or have a flu-like illness.[1] Loin pain can occur and acute pyelonephritis may be wrongly assumed to be the diagnosis.[56] Meningitis is extremely rare during pregnancy, although this is the most common presentation of listeriosis in other at-risk groups.[57] Placental transfer causes amnionitis, which usually results in spontaneous septic abortion, stillbirth or premature birth of an infected child.[56,57] The infected pre-term fetus may pass meconium and the diagnosis should be considered when liquor is meconium stained at less than 34 weeks gestation. Mortality rates are high in infected newborn infants. Complications include meningitis, encephalitis, pneumonia, conjunctivitis and thrombocytopenia with petechiae.[55]

A pregnant woman with unexplained fever for more than 48 hours, especially if followed by miscarriage or premature labour, should have blood sent for culture.[55] In the infant, cultures should be carried out if there has been maternal febrile illness during or immediately before delivery, if meconium staining of liquor is present or if signs of sepsis or meningitis develop. Expelled products of conception should also be cultured.[1]

If infection is diagnosed during pregnancy, the recommended treatment is IV ampicillin 6 g daily for two weeks.[58] In severely ill patients, gentamicin is usually added.[57] Intravenous erythromycin 4 g daily is an alternative for those allergic to penicillin, but is probably less effective and antagonism occurs if used in combination with gentamicin.[57,58]

Advice regarding prevention is to:

* avoid soft cheeses, pâtés and undercooked meats
* thoroughly wash raw vegetables before eating them
* avoid unpasteurised milk
* observe 'use by' date
* ensure that reheated food is piping hot all the way through.

Toxoplasmosis

Toxoplasma gondii is a protozoan parasite that has a sexual cycle in cats and an asexual cycle in other animal hosts such as humans. Infection occurs following ingestion of the parasite after handling contaminated soil or cat litter, eating poorly washed vegetables and fruit or eating undercooked infected meat. Infection is usually asymptomatic, although a glandular fever-like illness or cervical lymphadenopathy can occur. Serious disease, however, can result from congenital infection or infection in somebody with impaired immunity.

Over 20% of pregnant women have evidence of previous infection by toxoplasma.[59] It is estimated that in the UK acute maternal infection occurs in two per 1000 pregnancies or 1200 pregnancies each year.[59,60] Following acute maternal infection there is a 30–40% risk of congenital infection, with risk of infection increasing and severity of disease decreasing with the length of the pregnancy.[61-63] It is estimated that there should be about 400–500 congenital infections per year in the UK, of which 32–40 would be severe.[59] The actual number reported is much less with only about 13 cases of congenital infection reported annually.[1] It is likely that under-reporting occurs and that many asymptomatic cases are missed who are at risk of developing chorioretinitis later on in life.

Congenital infection early in pregnancy may result in miscarriage, stillbirth or severe neurological and eye disease in those that survive. The classic triad is hydrocephalus, intracranial calcification and chorioretinitis. Congenital infection in the second and third trimesters usually results in mild or subclinical disease at birth. However, progressive complications can develop as the child gets older, with seizures, mental handicap, spasticity, microcephaly or hydrocephalus, intracranial calcification, hearing loss and blindness.[64] Overall, it is estimated that 5–20% of live born infected infants will have permanent sequelae from toxoplasma infection.[62]

In the mother, infection is confirmed by seroconversion or by a significant rise in toxoplasma-specific IgG. High titre of specific IgG, or the presence of specific IgM, is very suggestive of active infection but is not diagnostic.[65] Prenatal testing to detect fetal infection involves ultrasound to try and detect signs of infection, such as hydrocephalus or cerebral calcification, and cordocentesis with testing of fetal blood for specific IgM. DNA amplification tests of amniotic fluid are also becoming available.[8] In the newborn infant, a positive IgM or persistence of specific IgG is diagnostic.[61] The absence of IgM does not exclude the diagnosis as the IgM response may be waning by the time of birth. Examination and culture of the placenta is occasionally useful.

The low incidence of congenital toxoplasmosis does not justify routine prenatal screening in the UK, although there is debate about this.[59,60,62,65,66] Some countries with higher incidence, e.g. France, have national prenatal screening programmes.

There is uncertainty about how effective current treatments are in preventing congenital infection.[67] Treatment of maternal infection with spiramycin, a macrolide antibiotic, possibly reduces the risk of congenital infection occurring by over 50%, although it does not reduce the severity of congenital infection.[60] Severity of infection may be reduced by combination therapy with pyrimethamine plus sulphadiazine, alternating monthly with spiramycin until delivery; therefore further tests to establish whether the fetus is infected should be considered.[60,62,63] In the UK, spiramycin is only available on a named-patient basis from IDIS. Pyrimethamine is a folate antagonist, and although there are no reports of fetal malformations associated with its use, folic acid is usually given with it.[44,68] There is a theoretical risk that sulphadiazine may cause kernicterus if given near term, due to displacement of protein-bound bilirubin; there is no evidence, however, of this being a problem in practice.[68]

Termination of pregnancy might be discussed if fetal infection is confirmed. However, it is difficult to estimate the risk of a child being symptomatic if the pregnancy is allowed to continue. In France, termination is only encouraged if maternal infection occurred early in pregnancy and there is evidence of fetal infection, or if there is ultrasound evidence of severe toxoplasmosis-related damage.[65]

Congenitally infected infants are treated with pyrimethamine, sulphadiazine and folic acid for at least one year, as this reduces the risk of progressive disease and can lead to improvement in some symptomatic infants.[64] Treatment regimes vary and are still being developed and consultation with tertiary specialist services is advised.

Although effectiveness has not been validated, the usual advice to try and avoid infection is:

- avoid cat litter
- avoid eating undercooked meat
- wear gloves or wash hands thoroughly after handling raw meat, and keep cutting boards and utensils thoroughly clean
- wear gloves when gardening
- wash vegetables thoroughly before eating them and, if handling raw vegetables, wear gloves or wash hands thoroughly afterwards.

Malaria

Malaria is a parasitic illness caused by *plasmodium* protozoa and is prevalent throughout tropical and subtropical areas of the world. Infection occurs following a bite from an infected *Anopheles* mosquito. Approximately 2000 cases are imported into the UK each year; about half of these are due to *Plasmodium falciparum*, and an average of seven cases die.[69] Malaria is especially hazardous during pregnancy, particularly when due to *Plasmodium falciparum*, probably due to altered immune responses.[70–72] Malaria in pregnancy can cause severe maternal anaemia, maternal and neonatal death, intrauterine growth retardation, miscarriage, stillbirth or premature delivery.[71,73] Congenital malaria is rare, and is more likely to occur following infection of non-immune pregnant women.[73] In view of the risks, pregnant women should ideally avoid travel to malaria-endemic areas, especially areas with drug-resistant *Plasmodium falciparum* malaria.[74]

Chemoprophylaxis of malaria throughout pregnancy is vital for all women visiting malaria-endemic areas. Strict attention should also be paid to personal protection measures against mosquito bites, such as the use of mosquito nets and mosquito repellents. Chloroquine and proguanil are safe in pregnancy; chemoprophylaxis should start one week before entering a malaria-endemic area and continue for four weeks after leaving. Proguanil is a folate antagonist and therefore, in pregnancy, folic acid 5 mg daily should also be taken. Chloroquine is not recommended if there is a history of epilepsy. Resistance to these agents is an increasing problem.[68,72,73]

If travel to resistant *falciparum* areas is unavoidable, mefloquine or Maloprim (dapsone–pyrimethamine) are used and appear to be safe, although there are theoretical safety concerns.[68,72,73,75] Ideally they should be avoided in the first trimester. Folic acid, 5 mg daily, should be given to those taking Maloprim as pyrimethamine is a folate antagonist.[73] Mefloquine and chloroquine plus proguanil have similar risks of both non-serious and serious central nervous system toxicity, although mefloquine has received most adverse publicity.[76] Mefloquine is not recommended if there is a history of psychiatric disturbance or epilepsy. If used, it should be started two to three weeks prior to travel; this allows protective levels to be reached by the time of arrival at the destination and sufficient time to change treatment if adverse effects occur. Doxycycline is contraindicated due to the well-recognised risk from tetracyclines of deposition in growing bones and teeth.[44]

Breastfeeding is not contraindicated in mothers taking standard prophylactic doses of chloroquine or proguanil.[46,47] Small amounts of mefloquine pass into breast milk and although breastfeeding is not recommended it is unlikely to cause harm.[46] Pyrimethamine is safe to use, but enough dapsone may pass into breast milk to cause toxicity; use of Maloprim is therefore not advised while breastfeeding.[47,68]

If a pregnant woman needs to travel to a malaria endemic area, advice should be obtained from the Malaria Reference Laboratory (tel: 020 7927 2437) as recommendations are constantly changing. This especially applies if travel to chloroquine-resistant areas is intended. Other telephone advice line numbers can be obtained from the *British National Formulary*.[77] If a pregnant woman is thought to have malaria, expert advice should always be sought.

Genital infections

Vulvovaginal candidiasis (thrush)

Candida albicans is a yeast that causes vulvovaginal candidiasis; after bacterial vaginosis it is the most common form of vaginitis in the UK. Affected women usually complain of vaginal itch and discharge. It is particularly likely to occur in pregnancy and, although not a danger to the fetus, can cause considerable distress to the mother.[78] Diagnosis is confirmed by culture of vaginal swabs.

Treatment in pregnancy is with topical imidazoles. Clotrimazole, miconazole and econazole are safe and effective in pregnancy, with cure rates of over 80%.[79] Systemic absorption of topical imidazoles is negligible.[78] First trimester use is best avoided, however, unless the woman has a severe infection, due to theoretical concerns regarding possible effects on androgen synthesis.[78] Doses and duration of treatment are as in non-pregnancy. Topical nystatin is much less effective, with cure rates ranging from 14% to 50%, and is not recommended.[79] Experience with the use of oral antifungal agents is lacking and these should therefore be avoided.

Bacterial vaginosis

Bacterial vaginosis is the most common vaginal infection in women of reproductive age. Affected women mainly complain of an unpleasant vaginal smell and discharge, but many are asymptomatic.[80] It is characterised by a reduction in vaginal lactobacilli and an increase in *Gardnerella vaginalis*, anaerobic Gram-negative rods and *Mycoplasma hominis*. It is uncertain whether it can be sexually transmitted and whether treatment of the male partner reduces the risk of further infection.[81]

A diagnosis of bacterial vaginosis is made from the history, clinical examination and positive microscopy (small Gram-positive *Gardnerella* species, Gram-negative coccobacilli, curved rods and absence of lactobacilli). A less practical criteria is that three of the following must be present for the diagnosis to be made:[82]

- a grey homogenous vaginal discharge
- clue cells (vaginal epithelial cells heavily coated with bacilli) seen on microscopy
- pH of vaginal secretions ≥ 4.5
- positive amine test (a fishy odour on adding alkali to vaginal fluid).

The prevalence of bacterial vaginosis during pregnancy varies from 10–30%, but up to 50% clear spontaneously and new cases seldom develop after 16 weeks gestation.[82–84] Bacterial vaginosis in pregnancy is strongly associated with an increased risk of premature delivery and post-partum endometritis following Caesarean section.[81,85,86] Although treatment of bacterial vaginosis reduces the risk of premature birth, there is still debate about whether all affected pregnant women require treatment.[85,87] There is general agreement that symptomatic pregnant women should be treated, and that asymptomatic women found to have bacterial vaginosis should be treated if there is a history of premature birth in a previous pregnancy. Screening women with a history of premature birth and treating identified infection is advocated by some, although this is not standard practice in the UK.[84,85] Oral metronidazole 400 mg twice daily for seven days cures 80–90% of cases.[84] Metronidazole appears to be safe in pregnancy but because of the remote possibility of teratogenicity, high doses or use in the first trimester should be avoided if possible.[53,88] Topical vaginal treatment with metronidazole or clindamycin is as effective as oral therapy at clearing bacterial vaginosis and has the potential advantage of decreased systemic absorption, decreased fetal exposure and reduced side-effects.[84,89] It is uncertain, however, whether topical treatments are as effective at reducing the risk of premature delivery.[81,85]

Breastfeeding can continue if a mother is given oral metronidazole. It is estimated that less than 10% of the recommended daily therapeutic infant dose is delivered via breast milk.[90] However, single large doses should be avoided if possible as there are theoretical safety concerns.[47] Metronidazole in breast milk may taste unpleasant but feeding problems are unusual.

Trichomoniasis

Vaginitis due to the protozoan *Trichomonas vaginalis* is a common sexually transmitted disease. Infection classically presents with green-yellow frothy vaginal discharge, irritation of the vulval and urethra with pain and itching, painful sexual intercourse, and dysuria. Vaginal discharge is the most frequent complaint, but the classical appearance is only present in approximately 10% of women and many women have asymptomatic infection.[2] The diagnosis is usually made on the history and examination with microscopic examination of a wet preparation of vaginal secretions or isolation of the organism on culture. There is a lack of data on whether infection has an adverse effect on pregnancy.[91] Treatment is usually only recommended for symptomatic infection. Metronidazole (*see* bacterial vaginosis) is effective, with microbiological cure rates of more than 90% at seven days. It is recommended that partners also receive treatment.[92] Other sexually transmitted diseases frequently co-exist with trichomonas infection and should be excluded in all cases.

Group B streptococcal infection

Group B streptococcus (GBS) infection is the most common bacterial cause of morbidity and mortality among newborn infants.[93,94] Infection is transmitted to the infant from the colonised maternal vagina during delivery, although ascending infection is also thought to occur. Estimates of GBS colonisation rates among pregnant women range from 15% to 40%.[94,95] Less than 1% of infants born to colonised mothers develop disease. A study in Oxford showed an incidence of GBS infection of 0.9/1000 births.[96]

Infected infants usually present within the first 48 hours of life with severe sepsis. Figures from the United States suggest at least a 6% mortality rate despite treatment.[94] Published UK figures are significantly higher than this with a 19% mortality rate from definite infection, although some of this difference may be due to different case mix.[96] Late-onset disease, beyond seven days of life, is less common and has lower mortality.[93] Factors associated with early onset disease are listed in Box 11.2.

Box 11.2: Risk factors for early onset neonatal infection[94,97,98]

- Pre-term rupture of membranes (less than 37 weeks gestation)
- Premature birth (less than 37 weeks gestation)
- Prolonged rupture of membranes (greater than 18 hours before delivery)
- Maternal fever during labour (greater than 38°C)
- Group B streptococcus bacteriuria at any time during the pregnancy
- Previous infant born with GBS infection

Whether, when, and how to screen for GBS infection is a difficult issue. Vaginal and anorectal culture is poorly sensitive, with up to 30–50% of carriers missed.[94,98] A positive culture early in the third trimester has a predictive value for infection at delivery of only 67%.[94] Antepartum antibiotic therapy is of limited value due to high rates of GBS recurrence by the time of delivery.[94] The exception is women with GBS bacteriuria as eradication of infection decreases the risk of pre-term labour, although genital colonisation usually persists. Screening late in the third trimester decreases the chance of missing late infection, and culture-positive women are treated nearer term, with reduced risk of recurrence by the time of delivery. However, this misses premature births, which are at highest risk of GBS complications. Neonatal antibiotic treatment may prevent some cases of GBS, but more than 60% are already symptomatic at, or shortly after, birth and are at high risk of GBS complications.[97] Intrapartum antibiotics appear to be the best treatment currently available, although treatment needs to be started at least four hours before delivery.[93,99,100] Intrapartum screening is limited by the lack of a rapid, sensitive test. Selective intrapartum treatment of women with risk factors (Box 11.2) has been shown to be effective but fails to prevent 25–30% of cases of early-onset GBS infection.[98,99]

Due to these problems and the low incidence of early neonatal GBS infection in the UK, routine screening is not advised.[98] Intrapartum antibiotic prophylaxis should be offered to those with identifiable risk factors. A common regime is IV penicillin G, initially 3 g and then 1.5 g every four hours from the onset of labour or rupture of membranes until delivery. If allergic to penicillin, IV erythromycin is given.[94,98]

Following delivery, the baby should be carefully observed for signs of infection, and if this is suspected antibiotics started immediately while awaiting the results of investigations.

There is work on developing a GBS capsular polysaccharide vaccine for the active immunisation of pregnant women. Passive immunisation with IV immunoglobulin is ineffective.

Breastfeeding can be started immediately following birth. There is no need to wait for maternal serum antibiotic levels to drop, and there is no evidence that breastfeeding can pass GBS from a colonised mother to her baby.[47,98]

Chlamydia infection

Chlamydia trachomatis is the most common sexually transmitted infection in the UK, with prevalence rates of 5% or more in women.[101,102] It can present with vaginal discharge, pelvic pain, postcoital or intermenstrual bleeding, or dysuria, but is asymptomatic in about 70% of women.[1,102] It is a cause of pelvic inflammatory disease, ectopic pregnancy, chronic pelvic pain and infertility. It can be transmitted from an infected mother to her child during delivery and may result in ophthalmia neonatorum or pneumonitis. Of exposed infants, 15–25% develop moderate to severe conjunctivitis and 5–15% develop pneumonitis.[103] It has also been associated with premature delivery and intrauterine growth retardation.[1]

Chlamydia is not routinely screened for in pregnancy and most cases will be identified because of symptoms requiring vaginal examination and the taking of endocervical swabs. There are a number of different tests in use for the identification of chlamydia infection, with differing degrees of sensitivity and specificity. The traditional gold standard is culture of the organism, but sensitivity is only 60–65% when assessed against newer techniques such as amplified DNA tests.[101] There is currently research into the use of such tests to screen urine, therefore avoiding the need for an invasive examination.[102] If chlamydia is diagnosed, the possibility of other coexistent sexually transmitted diseases, especially gonorrhoea, should be considered. Liaison with specialist genitourinary services is recommended to provide counselling, contact tracing and to ensure full investigation and effective treatment.

The usual treatment in non-pregnancy for *Chlamydia trachomatis* infection is with a tetracycline. These are contraindicated in pregnancy due to deposition in growing bones and teeth and resultant risk of fetal abnormalities.[44] Erythromycin, 500 mg four times daily for seven days, produces a 90% microbiological cure rate. Amoxicillin, 500 mg three times daily for seven days, is probably just as effective and is associated with fewer side-effects.[101,103,104] Both erythromycin and amoxycillin have been extensively used in pregnancy, with no evidence of harm. Azithromycin and clindamycin are also effective, but experience with their use in pregnancy is limited and they should therefore not be used.[103] It is uncertain whether microbiological cure of maternal chlamydia infection results in reduced neonatal transmission and complications.[103]

Genital herpes

Genital herpes is caused by herpes simplex virus. About 75% of cases are due to herpes simplex virus type 2 (HSV-2) and the rest are due to herpes simplex virus type 1 (HSV-1). Prevalence of antibody to HSV-2 in women is approximately 12%, with up to 80% of these having asymptomatic or unrecognised disease.[105] In 1996, approximately 10 000 cases of first-attack genital herpes in women were reported from genitourinary clinics in England.[106] This number is likely to be considerably greater as many cases are not seen in clinics and are not reported.

During pregnancy, primary infection is rare.[107] Recurrent disease is more common, however, it is still unusual for a woman with genital herpes to have an outbreak during the last weeks of pregnancy. Asymptomatic shedding is common, whether or not clinical signs of infection are present.[108]

The diagnosis of genital herpes is frequently missed. Herpetic lesions are classically blistering and painful, but they often present as only a small fissure or raw area, a painless ulcer, a small area of erythema or an area of irritation with no visible abnormality. If in doubt it is best to do a herpes culture. This may be falsely negative, however, especially in recurrent disease where sensitivity is only about 40%.[14]

Neonatal herpes infection is serious but extremely rare, occurring in less than two per 100 000 live births.[109] Greatest risk to the fetus occurs with vaginal delivery during a primary infection, which is often asymptomatic, when about 40% of infants become infected.[107–109] Transmission rates are lowest for women who acquire herpes before pregnancy, with a risk of about 0.04% if there are no signs of an outbreak at delivery. Even if lesions are present the risk of transmission is still low (0.25–5%), probably because of transplacental transfer of maternal antibodies.[107] A small number of cases are acquired post-partum, usually HSV-1 infection from oro-labial herpes or herpetic whitlow.[107]

Neonatal herpes infection usually presents after the early postnatal period, with onset of symptoms 5–19 days after birth. It has a high mortality rate. Presenting features include skin or scalp rashes, fever, lethargy, seizures and respiratory distress. Vesicles are present in only 40% at presentation and some infants have no vesicles at any stage of the illness.[107]

Statements regarding the management of genital herpes in pregnancy have recently been published in the UK and are outlined in Boxes 11.3 and 11.4.[109]

Box 11.3:   Management of pregnant women with first episode genital herpes

First and second trimesters

- Consider treatment with aciclovir, especially if severe symptoms or impaired immunity. Known to shorten the duration and reduce the severity of symptoms as well as decrease the duration of viral shedding.
- Continuous aciclovir in the last four weeks of pregnancy may prevent recurrence at term and hence the need for delivery by Caesarean section.
- At term, management should be as per recurrent HSV (*see* Box 11.4).

Third trimester

- Caesarean section should be considered for all women, particularly those developing symptoms within six weeks of delivery, as the risk of viral shedding in labour is very high.
- If vaginal delivery is unavoidable, aciclovir treatment of mother and baby may be indicated.

Box 11.4:   Management of pregnant women with recurrent genital herpes

- Sequential cultures during late gestation to predict viral shedding at term are not indicated.
- Caesarean section to prevent neonatal herpes should not be performed in women who do not have genital lesions at delivery.
- Symptomatic recurrences of genital herpes during the third trimester will be brief; vaginal delivery is appropriate if no lesions are present at delivery.
- The benefits of obtaining specimens for culture at delivery in order to identify women who are asymptomatically shedding HSV are unproven.
- Management of women with genital lesions at onset of labour is usually delivery by Caesarean section. However, there is evidence that the risks of vaginal delivery for the fetus are small and must be set against the risks to the mother of Caesarean section.

Although aciclovir is not licensed for use in pregnancy, there is substantial experience of its use and to date there is no evidence of harm.[109,110] There is little information currently available regarding the use of other antivirals in pregnancy. Doses of aciclovir are the same as in non-pregnancy. If required, for a first episode of genital herpes the usual dose is 200 mg orally five times daily for five days. Suppressive therapy is 400 mg twice daily.

Breastfeeding is not contraindicated unless the mother has lesions around the nipples. Aciclovir is excreted in breast milk but is not thought to be harmful.[109]

Gonorrhoea

Gonorrhoea is a sexually transmitted infection caused by the Gram-negative diplococcus *Neisseria gonorrhoea*. The diagnosis should be suspected in a woman with an abnormal vaginal discharge and dysuria, or if there is a history of sexual contact with an infected person. Approximately half of infected women are asymptomatic.[1] Although national reported rates are low at 22–43 cases per 100 000, there are marked geographical variations within the UK, with rates as high as 138 per 100 000 women and 292 per 100 000 men in inner London.[111] These are reported from departments of genitourinary medicine, so actual numbers are likely to be higher.

Gonorrhoea in pregnancy is associated with premature rupture of membranes and premature delivery, and in the post-partum period with severe endometritis and pelvic infection.[112] Infection can be transmitted to the infant during delivery, with a 30–50% risk of ophthalmia neonatorum.[113] This presents in the first few days of life with a profuse, purulent conjunctival discharge and if untreated can result in blindness.

Culture and microscopy of endocervical and urethral swabs will identify 90% of cases.[114] Penicillin resistance is an increasing problem and should be excluded.

Treatment is usually with a single oral dose of amoxycillin 3 g plus probenecid 1 g, which achieves a microbiological cure rate greater than 90%. If there is a history of penicillin allergy, or if penicillin resistance is identified, an alternative is single-dose IM ceftriaxone 250 mg or IM spectinomycin 2 g. All these are approved for use in pregnancy, with no evidence of teratogenicity.[112,113] It is uncertain whether treatment reduces the risk of ophthalmia neonatorum or post-partum sepsis, although this would seem likely.

There is a high prevalence of genital chlamydia infection in women with gonorrhoea, ranging from 30–60%, and empirical treatment is advised in all cases (*see* p. 135).[112] As with all sexually transmitted diseases, liaison with specialist genitourinary medicine services is recommended to provide counselling, contact tracing and to ensure full investigation and effective treatment.

Syphilis

Syphilis is a sexually transmitted disease caused by the spirochaete *Treponema pallidum*. Transmission of infection from an infected woman to the fetus mainly occurs during the second and third trimesters.[115] The risk of the fetus becoming infected decreases the longer the mother has had syphilis, with few cases reported in late syphilis.[116] Overall, at least 75% of babies born to untreated women with syphilis are infected.[115]

The incidence of syphilis decreased dramatically following the introduction of penicillin after the Second World War; from a peak number of 27 761 annual cases in England and Wales in 1946 to less than 4000 cases in 1990.[115] In the UK, the incidence of syphilis has remained low. In the three years between 1994 to 1997, at least 139 pregnant women were diagnosed and treated for syphilis, with 121 of these detected by antenatal screening.[117] Thirty-one of these women had early syphilis, with a high risk of fetal transmission, and 17 cases of probable congenital syphilis were reported. Risk factors for infectious syphilis in pregnancy include living in London and the South East, belonging to an ethnic minority, and birth outside of the UK, particularly in a developing country.[117]

Untreated congenital infection may result in abortion, stillbirth or premature delivery. For those that survive, typical features are rash, condylomata lata, hepatosplenomegaly, jaundice, anaemia, nasal congestion ('snuffles'), osteochondritis, oedema, pseudoparalysis and linear scars around the angles of the mouth from healed mucocutaneous lesions.[118] These features may only develop several weeks after birth.

Diagnosis of syphilis is by serology, as the organism is extremely difficult to see on microscopy and cannot be cultured. In the UK, all women are screened early in pregnancy with the Venereal Disease Research Laboratory (VDRL) test, with confirmation of positive results with the more specific fluorescent treponemal antibody (FTA) test.[1]

Treatment should be discussed with a genitourinary medicine specialist. Contact tracing should not be forgotten. Penicillin is the treatment of choice, with erythromycin as a less effective alternative for patients with penicillin allergy.[116,119] Tetracyclines may be more effective than erythromycin but are not advised during pregnancy due to deposition in growing bones and teeth.[44,119] In the United States, if an infected pregnant woman is allergic to penicillin, desensitisation and subsequent treatment with penicillin is recommended.[120] Treatment regimes should be the same as in the non-pregnant patient and vary according to the stage of syphilis diagnosed.[119,120]

Following birth, the baby should be examined and serological tests carried out. Serology can remain positive for up to six weeks due to passive transfer of antibodies from the mother. Tests should therefore be repeated at six weeks and three months. A rising titre is diagnostic of persistent infection.[114] An infant whose mother was treated with erythromycin should have a course of penicillin to ensure adequate treatment.[114]

Table 11.2: Summary of infections covered in chapter (see text for full details)

Condition	Recommended treatment	Comments	Breastfeeding
Viral infections			
Rubella	No therapy.	Avoid contact with rubella. If non-immune give rubella vaccine post-partum.	Safe (including after rubella vaccination).
CMV	No therapy.	Low incidence of symptomatic congenital infection, but poor prognosis if present.	Avoid if infant is very premature, or treat milk to inactivate virus.
Varicella	VZIG to mother if in contact with chickenpox at less than 20 weeks gestation or within three weeks of expected delivery and non-immune. Consider aciclovir.	VZIG to neonate if maternal chickenpox develops up to five days prior to delivery or two days after.	Safe but avoid if lesions on nipples.
Parvovirus	No therapy.	Consider *in utero* transfusion or early delivery and transfusion, if hydrops fetalis.	Safe.
Hepatitis B	Combined passive-active immunisation of neonate.	Prevents carrier state in 90% of infants.	Safe.
HIV	Zidovudine.	Reduces the risk of the infant becoming infecting by more than 70%.	Not advised (doubles the risk of the infant becoming infected).
Bacterial and other infections			
Respiratory infections	Amoxycillin. Erythromycin. Cephalosporin.	Use full adult dose.	Safe.
Asymptomatic bacteriuria and urinary tract infection	Amoxycillin. Nitrofurantoin. Cephalexin.	Amoxycillin resistance is an increasing problem. Avoid nitrofurantoin if known or suspected G6PD deficiency.	Avoid nitrofurantoin if infant suspected to be G6PD deficient.
Listeriosis	Amoxycillin. Erythromycin.	Preventative measures are important.	

Table 11.2: continued

Condition	Recommended treatment	Comments	Breastfeeding
Malaria prophylaxis	Chloroquine. Proguanil. Mefloquine. Maloprim.	All pregnant women should ideally avoid travel to malarious areas, especially areas with resistant falciparum malaria. Folate supplements if proguanil or Maloprim taken.	Uncertainty regarding mefloquine but probably safe. Avoid Maloprim.

Genital infections

Condition	Recommended treatment	Comments	Breastfeeding
Candidiasis	Topical imidazoles.	Negligible systemic absorption, but ideally avoid in first trimester due to theoretical safety concerns.	Safe.
Bacterial vaginosis	Oral metronidazole.	Treat if symptomatic. Still debate whether treatment required if asymptomatic, but advised if history of premature birth in previous pregnancy.	Safe but may alter taste of milk.
Trichomoniasis	Oral metronidazole.	Treat if symptomatic.	Safe but may alter taste of milk.
Group B streptococcus	Intrapartum IV penicillin or erythromycin.	Controversy over risk factor assessment versus bacteriological screening.	Safe.
Genital herpes	Consider aciclovir if primary infection. Caesarean section if primary infection within six days of delivery date, or if recurrent disease and active lesions at time of delivery.	Debate over whether recurrent disease ever requires Caesarean section.	Safe.
Gonorrhoea	Single dose oral amoxycillin plus probenecid, or IM ceftriaxone or spectinomycin.	Greater than 90% cure rate.	Safe.
Syphilis	IM procaine penicillin. Oral erythromycin if penicillin allergic.	Standard course of treatment as in non-pregnancy, depending on stage of syphilis. Erythromycin less effective and not used in USA.	Safe.

Acknowledgements

Thanks to Dr Elizabeth Miller, consultant to the PHLS, for her many helpful comments. Also thanks to my colleagues Dr Helen Raison and Miss Kirsten Shearer.

References

1   Public Health Laboratory Service (1993) *TORCH Screening Reassessed: the laboratory investigation of congenital, perinatal and neonatal infection.* PHLS, London.

2   Wang MJ and Smaill F (1991) Infection in pregnancy. In *Effective Care in Pregnancy and Childbirth* (eds I Chalmers, M Enkin and M Kierse), pp. 534–64. Oxford University Press, Oxford.

3   Anonymous (1998) *Rubella laboratory reports, England and Wales, 1984–1996.* Laboratory reports to CDSC, 1998. PHLS Communicable Disease Surveillance Centre, London. Notes: http://www.phls.co.uk/cdsc/rub%2Dt05.htm

4   Miller E, Waight P, Gay N *et al.* (1997) The epidemiology of rubella in England and Wales before and after the 1994 measles and rubella vaccination campaign: 4th joint report from the PHLS and the National Congenital Rubella Surveillance Programme. *Comm Dis Rep.* **7**: R26–R32.

5   Miller E, Cradock-Watson JE and Pollock TM (1982) Consequences of confirmed maternal rubella at successive stages of pregnancy. *Lancet.* **2**: 781–4.

6   Enders G, Miller E, Nickerl-Pacher U and Cradock-Watson JE (1988) Outcome of confirmed periconceptional maternal rubella. *Lancet.* **i**: 1447.

7   Smithells RW, Sheppard S, Holzel H and Dickson A (1985) National Congenital Rubella Surveillance Programme 1 July 1971–30 June 1984. *BMJ Clin Res Ed.* **291**: 40–1.

8   Litwin CM and Hill HR (1997) Serologic and DNA-based testing for congenital and perinatal infections. *Ped Infect Dis J.* **16**: 1166–75.

9   Aboudy Y, Fogel A, Barnea B *et al.* (1997) Subclinical rubella re-infection during pregnancy followed by transmission of virus to the fetus. *J Infect.* **34**: 273–6.

10 Terry GM, Ho-Terry L, Warren RC *et al.* (1986) First trimester prenatal diagnosis of congenital rubella: a laboratory investigation. *BMJ Clin Res Ed.* **292**: 930–3.

11 Infectious Diseases and Immunisation Committee, Canadian Pediatric Society (1983) *Breastfeeding by Infected Mothers.* Notes: http://www.cps.ca/english/statements/ID/id83–02.htm

12 Nelson CT and Demmler GJ (1997) Cytomegalovirus infection in the pregnant mother, fetus, and newborn infant. *Clin Perinat.* **24**: 151–60.

13 Daniel Y, Gull I, Peyser MR and Lessing JB (1995) Congenital cytomegalovirus infection. *Eur J Obstet Gynecol Reprod Biol.* **63**: 7–16.

14 Scott LL, Hollier LM, Dias K (1997) Perinatal herpes virus infections. Herpes simplex, varicella and cytomegalovirus. *Infect Dis Clin North America.* **11**: 27–53.

15 Ramsay MEB, Miller E and Peckham CS (1991) Outcome of confirmed symptomatic congenital cytomegalovirus infection. *Arch Dis Child.* **66**: 1068–9.

16 Vochem M, Hamprecht K, Jahn G and Speer CP (1998) Transmission of cytomegalovirus to preterm infants through breast milk. *Ped Infect Dis J.* **17**: 53–8.

17 Infectious Disease and Immunisation Committee, CPS (1994) Chickenpox: prevention and treatment. *Can J Ped.* **1**: 88–93.

18 Seidman DS, Stevenson DK and Arvin AM (1996) Varicella vaccine in pregnancy. *BMJ.* **313**: 701–2.

19 Royal College of Obstetricians and Gynaecologists, UK (1997) *Chickenpox in Pregnancy.* Notes: http://www.rcog.org.uk/guidelines/chicken_pox.html

20 Nathwani D, Maclean A, Conway S and Carrington D (1998) Varicella infections in pregnancy and the newborn. A review prepared for the UK Advisory Group on Chickenpox on behalf of the British Society for the Study of Infection. *J Infect.* **36**: 59–71.

21 Enders G, Miller E, Cradock-Watson J *et al.* (1994) Consequences of varicella and herpes zoster in pregnancy: prospective study of 1739 cases. *Lancet.* **343**: 1548–51.

22 Ogilvie MM (1998) Antiviral prophylaxis and treatment in chickenpox. A review prepared for the UK Advisory Group on Chickenpox on behalf of the British Society for the Study of Infection. *J Infect.* **36**: 31–8.

23 Department of Health (1996) *Immunisation Against Infectious Disease.* The Stationery Office, London.

24 Anderson LJ (1987) Role of parvovirus B19 in human disease. *Ped Infect Dis J.* **6**: 711–18.

25 Harger JH, Adler SP, Koch WC and Harger GF (1998) Prospective evaluation of 618 pregnant women exposed to parvovirus B19: risks and symptoms. *Obstet Gynecol.* **91**: 413–420.

26 Miller E, Fairley CK, Cohen BJ and Seng C (1998) Immediate and long-term outcome of human parvovirus B19 infection in pregnancy. *Br J Obstet Gynaecol.* **105**: 174–8.

27 Gray ES, Anand A and Brown T (1986) Parvovirus infections in pregnancy [letter]. *Lancet.* **1**: 208.

28 Kinney JS, Anderson LJ, Farrar J *et al.* (1988) Risk of adverse outcomes of pregnancy after human parvovirus B19 infection. *J Infect Dis.* **157**: 663–7.

29 Rodis JF, Rodner C, Hansen AA *et al.* (1998) Long-term outcome of children following maternal human parvovirus B19 infection. *Obstet Gynecol.* **91**: 125–8.

30 Pastorek II JG (1995) Viral diseases. In *High Risk Pregnancy: management options* (eds DK James, PJ Steer, CP Weiner, B Gonik), pp. 481–507. WB Saunders Co Ltd, Philadelphia.

31 Fairley CK, Smoleniec JS, Caul OE and Miller E (1995) Observational study of effect of intrauterine transfusions on outcome of fetal hydrops after parvovirus B19 infection. *Lancet.* **346**: 1335–7.

32 Rodis JF, Borgida AF, Wilson M *et al.* (1998) Management of parvovirus infection in pregnancy and outcomes of hydrops: a survey of members of the Society of Perinatal Obstetricians. *Am J Obstet Gynecol.* **179**: 985–8.

33 Development & Evaluation Committee (DEC), The Wessex Institute for Health Service Research & Development (1996) *Screening for Hepatitis B in Pregnancy.* **Report 61**: 1–33.

34 Infectious Disease and Immunisation Committee (CPS) (1986) Hepatitis B: update on perinatal management. *Can Med Assoc J.* **134**: 883–6.

35 Stevens CE, Toy PT, Tong MJ *et al.* (1985) Perinatal hepatitis B virus transmission in the United States. Prevention by passive-active immunisation. *JAMA.* **253**: 1740–5.

36   Anonymous (1997) *Prevalence of HIV in England and Wales, 1996. Unlinked anonymous HIV seroprevalence monitoring programme in England and Wales. Summary report from the Unlinked Anonymous Surveys Steering Group.* Department of Health, Public Health Laboratory Service, Institute of Child Health, London. Notes: http: //www.open.gov.uk/doh/pub/doc/doh/hiv.pdf

37   Anonymous (1998) Royal College of Paediatrics and Child Health, Royal College *Reducing mother to child transmission of HIV infection in the United Kingdom. Recommendations of an intercollegiate working party for enhancing voluntary confidential HIV testing in pregnancy.* of Obstetricians and Gynaecologists, Public Health Laboratory Service. Notes: http: //www.open.gov.uk/cdsc/rcpch.pdf

38   Brocklehurst P (1998) Interventions aimed at decreasing the risk of mother-to-child transmission of HIV infection (Cochrane Review). *The Cochrane Library.* Issue **3**. Update Software, Oxford.

39   Connor EM, Sperling RS, Gelber R *et al.* (1994) Reduction of maternal-infant transmission of human immunodeficiency virus type 1 with zidovudine treatment. Pediatric AIDS Clinical Trials Group Protocol 076 Study Group. *NEJM.* **331**: 1173–80.

40   Anonymous (1997) Major advances in the treatment of HIV-1 infection. *Drug Therap Bull.* **35**: 29.

41   Dennison B, Kennedy J, Tilling K *et al.* (1998) Feasibility of named antenatal HIV screening in an inner city population. *Aids Care.* **10**: 259–65.

42   Department of Health (1999) *Reducing Mother to Baby Transmission of HIV.* Health Service Circular 1999/183.

43   Clinton MJ, Niederman MS and Matthay RA (1992) Maternal pulmonary disorders complicating pregnancy. In *Medicine of the Fetus and Mother* (eds E Albert Reece, JC Hobbins, MJ Mahoney, Petrie RH), pp 955–81. JB Lippincott Co, St Louis.

44   Gilstrap III LC and Little BB (1998) Antimicrobial agents during pregnancy. In *Drugs and Pregnancy* (ed Anon), pp 45–75. Chapman & Hall, London.

45   Anonymous (1998) Antibiotic treatment of adults with chest infection in general practice. *Drug Therap Bull.* **36**: 68–72.

46   Anderson PO (1991) Drug use during breast-feeding. *Clin Pharm.* **10**: 594–624.

47   Bennett PN and WHO Working Group (1988) *Drugs and Human Lactation.* Elsevier, Amsterdam.

48   Smaill F (1998) Antibiotic vs no treatment for asymptomatic bacteriuria in pregnancy (Cochrane Review). *The Cochrane Library.* Issue **3**. Update Software, Oxford.

49   Tan JS and File TM Jr (1992) Treatment of bacteriuria in pregnancy [published erratum appears in *Drugs* (1993) **46**(2): 268]. *Drugs.* **44**: 972–980.

50   Bint AJ and Hill D (1994) Bacteriuria of pregnancy: an update on significance, diagnosis and management. *J Antimicrob Chemo.* **33**(Suppl A): 93–7.

51   Villar J, Lydon-Rochelle MT and Gülmezoglu AM (1998) Duration of treatment for asymptomatic bacteriura during pregnancy (Cochrane Review). *The Cochrane Library.* Issue **3**. Update Software, Oxford.

52   Ben David S, Einarson T, Ben David Y *et al.* (1995) The safety of nitrofurantoin during the first trimester of pregnancy: meta-analysis. *Funda Clin Pharma.* **9**: 503–7.

53   Korzeniowski OM (1995) Antibacterial agents in pregnancy. *Infect Dis Clin North America.* **9**: 639–51.

54   Anonymous (1998) *Human listeriosis cases England and Wales, 1983–97. Laboratory reports to CDSC, PHLS, Food Hygiene Laboratory, 1998.* PHLS Communicable Disease Surveillance Centre, London. Notes: http: //www.phls.co.uk/cdsc/list-t01.htm

55 Wilkinson P (1992) Uncommon infections: listeriosis. *Prescrib J.* **32**: 26–31.

56 Craig S, Permezel M, Doyle L *et al.* (1996) Perinatal infection with Listeria monocytogenes. *Aust NZ J Obstet Gynaecol.* **36**: 286–90.

57 Lorber B (1997) Listeriosis. *Clin Infect Dis.* **24**: 1–9.

58 Jones EM and MacGowan AP (1995) Antimicrobial chemotherapy of human infection due to Listeria monocytogenes. *Eur J Clin Micro Infect Dis.* **14**: 165–75.

59 Joynson DHM (1992) Epidemiology of toxoplasmosis in the UK. *Scan J Infect Dis.* **Suppl 84**: 65–9.

60 Holliman RE (1995) Congenital toxoplasmosis: prevention, screening and treatment. *J Hosp Infect.* **130**(Suppl): 179–90.

61 Mombro M, Perathoner C, Leone A *et al.* (1995) Congenital toxoplasmosis: 10-year follow up. *Eur J Peds.* **154**: 635–9.

62 Eskild A, Oxman A, Magnus P *et al.* (1996) Screening for toxoplasmosis in pregnancy: what is the evidence of reducing a health problem? *J Med Screen.* **3**: 188–94.

63 Lynfield R and Guerina NG (1997) Toxoplasmosis. *Ped Rev.* **18**: 75–83.

64 Roizen N, Swisher CN, Stein MA *et al.* (1995) Neurologic and developmental outcome in treated congenital toxoplasmosis. *Ped.* **95**: 11–20.

65 Hall SM (1992) Congenital toxoplasmosis. *BMJ.* **305**: 291–7.

66 Lappalainen M, Sintonen H, Koskiniemi M *et al.* (1995) Cost-benefit analysis of screening for toxoplasmosis during pregnancy. *Scan J Infect Dis.* **27**: 265–72.

67 Wallon M, Liou C, Garner P and Peyron F (1999) Congenital toxoplasmosis: systematic review of evidence of efficacy of treatment in pregnancy. *BMJ.* **318**: 1511–14.

68 Phillips-Howard PA and Wood D (1996) The safety of antimalarial drugs in pregnancy. *Drug Safety.* **14**: 131–45.

69 Anonymous (1998) *AIDS/HIV Quarterly Surveillance Tables: UK data to end June 1998.* Public Health Laboratory Service, AIDS Centre, Scottish Centre for Infection & Environmental Health. Notes: http://www.open.gov.uk/cdsc/q0698.pdf

70 Bruce-Chwatt LJ (1983) Malaria and pregnancy. *BMJ Clin Res Ed.* **286**: 1457–8.

71 Mutabingwa TK (1994) Malaria and pregnancy: epidemiology, pathophysiology and control options. *Acta Tropica.* **57**: 239–54.

72 Bradley DJ and Warhurst DC (1997) Guidelines for the prevention of malaria in travellers from the United Kingdom: PHLS Malaria Reference Laboratory, London School of Hygiene and Tropical Medicine. *Communicable Disease Report (CDR Review).* **7**: R137–R152.

73 Silver HM (1997) Malarial infection during pregnancy. *Infect Dis Clin North America.* **11**: 99–107.

74 Ahmed A, Cerilli LA and Sanchez PJ (1998) Congenital malaria in a pre-term neonate: case report and review of the literature. *Am J Perinat.* **15**: 19–22.

75 Vanhauwere B, Maradit H and Kerr L (1998) Post-marketing surveillance of prophylactic mefloquine (Lariam) use in pregnancy. *Am J Trop Med Hyg.* **58**: 17–21.

76 Anonymous (1998) Mefloquine and malaria prophylaxis. *Drug Thera Bull.* **36**: 22.

77 British Medical Association, Royal Pharmaceutical Society of Great Britain (1998) *British National Formulary.* BMA, RPS, London.

78 Sullivan C and Smith LG Jr (1993) Management of vulvovaginitis in pregnancy. *Clin Obstet Gynecol.* **36**: 195–205.

79 Reef SE, Levine WC, McNeil MM *et al.* (1995) Treatment options for vulvovaginal candidiasis. *Clin Infect Dis.* **20**(Suppl 1): S80–S90.

80 Mead PB (1993) Epidemiology of bacterial vaginosis. *Am J Obstet Gynecol.* **169**: 446–9.

81 Anonymous (1998) Management of bacterial vaginosis. *Drug Ther Bull.* **36**: 33–5.

82 MacDermott RI (1995) Bacterial vaginosis. *Br J Obstet Gynaecol.* **102**: 92–4.

83 Hay PE, Morgan DJ, Ison CA *et al.* (1994) A longitudinal study of bacterial vaginosis during pregnancy. *Br J Obstet Gynaecol.* **101**: 1048–53.

84 Society of Obstetricians and Gynaecologists of Canada (1997) *Bacterial vaginosis: clinical practice guidelines. Committee opinion No.14.* Notes: http: //sogc.medical.org/ sogc_docs/public/guidelines/baclast.htm

85 McGregor JA, French JI, Parker R *et al.* (1995) Prevention of premature birth by screening and treatment for common genital tract infections: results of a prospective controlled evaluation. *Am J Obstet Gynecol.* **173**: 157–67.

86 Watts DH, Krohn MA, Hillier SL and Eschenbach DA (1990) Bacterial vaginosis as a risk factor for post-cesarean endometritis. *Obstet Gynecol.* **75**: 52–8.

87 Morales WJ, Schorr S and Albritton J (1994) Effect of metronidazole in patients with pre-term birth in preceding pregnancy and bacterial vaginosis: a placebo-controlled, double-blind study. *Am J Obstet Gynecol.* **171**: 345–7.

88 Burtin P, Taddio A, Ariburnu O *et al.* (1995) Safety of metronidazole in pregnancy: a meta-analysis. *Am J Obstet Gynecol.* **172**: 525–9.

89 Hillier SL, Lipinski C, Briselden AM and Eschenbach DA (1993) Efficacy of intravaginal 0.75% metronidazole gel for the treatment of bacterial vaginosis. *Obstet Gynecol.* **81**: 963–7.

90 Passmore CM, McElnay JC, Rainey EA and D'Arcy PF (1988) Metronidazole excretion in human milk and its effect on the suckling neonate. *Br J Clin Pharma.* **26**: 45–51.

91 Gulmezoglu AM (1998) Trichomoniasis treatment during pregnancy. *The Cochrane Library.* Update Software, Oxford.

92 Wendel PJ and Wendel GD Jr (1993) Sexually transmitted diseases in pregnancy. *Sem Perinat.* **17**: 443–51.

93 Ohlsson A and Myhr TL (1994) Intrapartum chemoprophylaxis of perinatal group B streptococcal infections: a critical review of randomised controlled trials. *Am J Obstet Gynecol.* **170**: 910–17.

94 Anonymous (1996) Prevention of perinatal group B streptococcal disease: a public health perspective. Centers for Disease Control and Prevention [published erratum appears in *Morb Mortal Wkly Rep* (1996) **45**(31): 679]. *MMWR – Morb Mort Wkly Rep.* **45**: 1–24.

95 Regan JA, Klebanoff MA and Nugent RP (1991) The epidemiology of group B streptococcal colonisation in pregnancy. Vaginal Infections and Prematurity Study Group. *Obstet Gynecol.* **77**: 604–10.

96 Moses LM, Heath PT, Wilkinson AR *et al.* (1998) Early onset group B streptococcus neonatal infection in Oxford 1985–96. *Arch Dis Child (Fetal Neonatal Ed).* **79**: F148–F149.

97 Society of Obstetricians and Gynaecologists of Canada, Canadian Paediatric Society (1994) *National consensus statement on the prevention of early-onset group B streptococcal infections in the newborn, No. 7.* SOGC, CPS. Notes: http: //sogc.medical. org/sogc_docs/public/guidelines/earlyon.htm

98 Anonymous (1997) *Group B streptococcus: the facts.* Group B Strep Support. Notes: http: //www.gbs.org.uk/

99   Allen UD, Navas L and King SM (1993) Effectiveness of intrapartum penicillin prophylaxis in preventing early-onset group B streptococcal infection: results of a meta-analysis. *CMAJ.* **149**: 1659–65.

100 Smaill F (1998) Intrapartum antibiotics for group B streptococcal colonisation (Cochrane Review). *The Cochrane Library.* Issue **3**. Update Software, Oxford.

101 Anonymous (1998) *The 4th Bandolier Conference: Chlamydia.* Notes: http://www.jr2.ox.ac.uk/bandolier/bandopubs/bandocon4/chlamyd.html

102 Anonymous (1998) *Summary and conclusions of CMO's Expert Advisory Group on Chlamydia trachomatis.* Department of Health, London. Notes: http://www.open.gov.uk/doh/chlamyd.htm

103 Brocklehurst P and Rooney G (1998) The treatment of genital *Chlamydia trachomatis* infection in pregnancy (Cochrane Review). *The Cochrane Library.* Issue **3**. Update Software, Oxford.

104 Turrentine MA and Newton ER (1995) Amoxicillin or erythromycin for the treatment of antenatal chlamydial infection: a meta-analysis. *Obstet Gynecol.* **86**: 1021–5.

105 Cowan FM, Johnson AM, Ashley R *et al.* (1994) Antibody to herpes simplex virus type 2 as serological marker of sexual lifestyle in populations. *BMJ.* **309**: 1325–9.

106 Hughes G and Catchpole M (1998) Surveillance of sexually transmitted infections in England and Wales. *Eur Comm Dis Bull.* **3**: 61–5.

107 New Zealand Herpes Foundation (1996) *Guidelines for the management of genital herpes in New Zealand.* Notes: http://www.nzhealth.co.nz/herpes/guide/index.html

108 Brown ZA, Benedetti J, Ashley R *et al.* (1991) Neonatal herpes simplex virus infection in relation to asymptomatic maternal infection at the time of labor. *NEJM.* **324**: 1247–52.

109 Smith JR, Cowan FM and Munday P (1998) The management of herpes simplex virus infection in pregnancy. *Br J Obstet Gynaecol.* **105**: 255–60.

110 Anonymous (1993) Pregnancy outcomes following systemic prenatal aciclovir exposure: 1 June 1984–30 June 1993. *Morb Mortal Wkly Rep.* **42**: 806–9.

111 Low N, Daker-White G, Barlow D and Pozniak AL (1997) Gonorrhoea in inner London: results of a cross sectional study. *BMJ.* **314**: 1719–23.

112 Cavenee MR, Farris JR, Spalding TR *et al.* (1993) Treatment of gonorrhea in pregnancy. *Obstet Gynecol.* **81**: 33–8.

113 Brocklehurst P (1998) Treatment of gonorrhoea in pregnancy (Cochrane Review). *The Cochrane Library.* Issue **3**. Update Software, Oxford.

114 Adler MW, Gilson R, Goldmeier D *et al.* (1995) *ABC of Sexually Transmitted Diseases.* BMJ Publishing Group, London.

115 Walker GJA (1998) Antibiotic treatment for pregnant women infected with syphilis (Cochrane Review). *The Cochrane Library.* Issue **3**. Update Software, Oxford.

116 Adler MW (1984) ABC of sexually transmitted diseases: pregnancy and the neonate. *BMJ Clin Res Ed.* **288**: 624–7.

117 Hurtig A-K, Nicoll A, Carne C *et al.* (1998) Syphilis in pregnant women and their children in the United Kingdom: results from national clinician reporting surveys 1994–7. *BMJ.* **317**: 1617–19.

118 Ratcliffe L, Nicoll A, Carrington D *et al.* (1998) Reference laboratory surveillance of syphilis in England and Wales: 1994 to 1996. *Comm Dis Pub Health.* **1**: 14–21.

119 Rolfs RT (1995) Treatment of syphilis: 1993. *Clin Infect Dis.* **20**(Suppl 1): S23–S38.

120 Anonymous (1998) Guidelines for the treatment of sexually transmitted diseases. *Morb Mortal Wkly Rep.* **47**: 1–118.

CHAPTER TWELVE

Endocrine disorders

Helen Seymour and Kathryn Pughe

Diabetes

Introduction

About two to three women per thousand of reproductive age have diabetes before conception. Type I diabetes mellitus, also known as insulin-dependent diabetes mellitus (IDDM), complicates less than 0.5% of pregnancies.[1] Type II diabetes mellitus, or non-insulin dependent diabetes mellitus (NIDDM), is less common in the age group likely to become pregnant. When glucose intolerance is first identified during a pregnancy this is called gestational diabetes, which complicates approximately 5% of pregnancies.[2] Women with a history of gestational diabetes are likely to develop Type II DM.[3]

Possible adverse fetal effects

Fetal and neonatal death occurs in about 2–4% of Type I DM pregnancies in specialist centres[1] compared with about 1.2% in the general population.[4] Poor fetal outcome may be slightly more likely in non-specialist settings – one study showed a 4.5% rate of fetal and neonatal death in the absence of specialist regional guidelines.[4] Stillbirth incidence is greatest at 36 weeks gestation. The risk of this is particularly high if there is a history of poor glycaemic control, maternal vascular disease, ketoacidosis, pre-eclampsia or fetal macrosomia. Major congenital anomalies occur in 5–10% of Type I DM pregnancies (between two and four times higher than in normal pregnancies). Risk factors for major congenital anomaly include poor diabetic control, both pre-conception and during pregnancy, duration of Type I DM greater than 10 years and diabetic vasculopathy. Anomalies include cardiac malformations

(4% of diabetic vs 0.08% of normal pregnancies), most commonly ventricular septal defects, transposition of the great vessels and coarctation of the aorta; neural tube defect (2% vs 0.2%); caudal regression syndrome in 0.5%, which includes sacral agenesis and phocomelic diabetic embryopathy; and renal and gastrointestinal defects.[1] In the Casson study the overall malformation rate of total births was 9.7% in the Type I DM patients compared with 1.0% in the general population; of these, 40% were cardiovascular. Neonatal jaundice has been reported in 53% of pregnancies complicated by Type I DM and 38% of pregnancies with gestational diabetes.[5]

Good metabolic control is the cornerstone of management of the pregnant diabetic. Pregnancies should be planned and pre-conception counselling offered. The risk of malformation is directly related to the haemoglobin A_1 concentration at the time of conception, therefore pregnancy should be deferred until good metabolic control has been maintained for some time.[6] Care should be delivered by a multidisciplinary team, including an obstetrician, diabetologist, diabetes specialist nurse, midwife and dietician.[7]

Hypertension should be evaluated and treated prior to pregnancy to reduce the progression of diabetic nephropathy[8] (*see* Chapter 6).

Good metabolic control prior to and during pregnancy improves outcome.

Drug treatment

Insulin-dependent diabetes

Expert dietary advice from a dietician is essential. Snacks should be eaten between meals and at bedtime to reduce the incidence of ketogenesis. Additional calorie intake should be in the form of complex carbohydrate, and protein supplementation may also be required.

Regular home blood glucose monitoring is necessary if good diabetic control is to be achieved. Insulin does not cross the placenta but metabolic disturbances due to excess or lack of insulin will affect the fetus. Hypoglycaemic attacks are more common during pregnancy. Tight glycaemic control is usually achieved with a combination of separate soluble and medium- or long-acting insulins as this provides better flexibility than fixed combination products. This is either given as a twice-daily combination of short- and long-acting insulin or as multiple daily injections of short-acting insulin prior to meals with a long acting insulin at bedtime. It is outside the scope of this book to give detailed guidance on individual insulin regimes, expert advice from a diabetologist should be obtained.

Human rather than animal insulin should be used. Human insulin has been shown to reduce the incidence of macrosomia and to provide better glycaemic control than animal insulins.[7]

- **Use human rather than animal insulin.**
- **Use separate soluble and intermediate/long-acting preparations.**
- **Liaise with dietician to optimise nutrition.**

Non-insulin-dependent diabetes

Patients controlled on oral hypoglycaemic agents prior to pregnancy should be converted to an insulin regime, preferably as part of pre-pregnancy planning and certainly in early pregnancy. There is no evidence that metformin or sulphonylureas are teratogenic. However, metformin may be associated with growth retardation and hyperbilirubinaemia. Sulphonylureas cross the placenta and may cause hyperinsulinaemia and macrosomia in the fetus.[7,9]

- **Convert patients on oral hypoglycaemic agents to human insulin as soon as possible.**

Gestational diabetes

Gestational diabetes can generally be managed by restricting refined carbohydrates. Exercise is recommended in women without medical or obstetric complications.[10] Maternal glucose levels should be monitored carefully throughout the third trimester. If, despite dietary management, fasting plasma glucose levels exceed 5.8 mmol/L, or postprandial levels exceed 6.7 mmol/L, then human insulin therapy should be started.[5,7]

- **Start insulin in women with significant fasting or post prandial hyperglycaemia.**

Hypoglycaemia

By increasing glycaemic control, hypoglycaemia is more likely to occur due to increased sensitivity to insulin, especially in the first trimester.[11] Women with hyperemesis are at higher risk of hypoglycaemia. Patients and their relatives must be made aware of the risk of nocturnal hypoglycaemia; clinical evidence includes nightmares, headaches upon waking, night sweats, hypothermia, tingling in the extremities and morning lassitude.[11]

Occasional hypoglycaemia is a much lower risk to the fetus than persistent hyperglycaemia. Hypoglycaemia can be treated conventionally with a glass of milk, which can be repeated in 15 minutes if symptoms remain. Severe hypoglycaemia should be treated with glucagon injection.[7,12,13]

Treat hypoglycaemia conventionally.

Diabetic ketoacidosis

Ketoacidosis affects about 1% of diabetic pregnancies and leads to a 20% chance of fetal loss. It is more common in Type I DM than in Type II DM or gestational diabetes. Causes include hyperemesis, infections, corticosteroid use, insulin-pump failure and beta-sympathomimetic agents. Ketoacidosis occurs mainly in the first trimester and may occur with minimal hyperglycaemia.

Management of diabetic ketoacidosis in pregnancy is the same as in the non-pregnant state, with particular emphasis on correcting maternal acidosis as quickly as possible.[1,5]

- **Diabetic ketoacidosis is associated with significant fetal mortality.**
- **There may be minimal hyperglycaemia.**
- **Correct metabolic acidosis conventionally.**

Management during delivery

If there are no complications the pregnancy can continue to 39–40 weeks gestation. There are many regimes for the management of diabetes during labour. An IV infusion of dextrose plus potassium should be set up together with a separate infusion of soluble insulin, and local policy guidelines followed (a specimen regime is outlined in Box 12.1). Blood glucose should be monitored hourly and tailored to individual requirements. For patients who are nil-by-mouth, other electrolyte requirements, particularly sodium and chloride, should not be neglected. The aim is to maintain euglycaemia, especially in the second stage of labour, to minimise the risk of neonatal hypoglycaemia. Immediately after delivery of the baby and placenta, insulin requirements fall rapidly and the insulin content of the dextrose infusion should be halved or, in women with gestational diabetes, stopped. It is usual to restart pre-pregnancy insulin regimes soon after delivery.[7,12]

Box 12.1:   A specimen regime for diabetes management in labour

Start an infusion of 500 mL 10% dextrose plus 10 mmol potassium chloride. Add 50 units soluble insulin to 50 mL 0.9% saline and give via an infusion pump according to the following sliding scale:

Blood glucose	*Change to*
>13.0 mmol/L	6 units/h and check blood glucose every 30 minutes
10.1–13.0 mmol/L	3 units/h
8.1–10.0 mmol/L	2 units/h
4.1–8.0 mmol/L	1 unit/h
2.0–4.0 mmol/L	0.3 units/h plus 100 mL 10% dextrose
<2.0 mmol/L	0.3 units/h plus 150 mL 10% dextrose

Breastfeeding

Breastfeeding should be encouraged. A high fluid and calcium intake should be maintained and insulin administered in the usual way. Carbohydrate snacks prior to feeding will reduce the incidence of hypoglycaemia.

Metformin is believed to be excreted in breast milk in fairly high concentrations and should be avoided. Tolbutamide is excreted in breast milk; the American Academy of Pediatrics note that there is a possibility of jaundice in the nursing infant but considers tolbutamide to be compatible with breastfeeding. There is also a concern that both metformin and tolbutamide may cause neonatal hypoglycaemia; if used, the infant should be closely monitored, with regular blood glucose monitoring. The other sulphonylureas should be avoided; they are excreted in breast milk and there have been isolated reports of hypoglycaemia in the infant.[14,15] If patients with Type II DM continue to require drug therapy after birth then they should be maintained on insulin until breastfeeding is stopped. Obviously the doses of insulin required will be lower than that required during pregnancy.

Summary

Table 12.1:   Management of maternal diabetes

Condition	Management recommendations
Insulin-dependent diabetes	Pre-pregnancy planning. Maintain tight metabolic control using human soluble and intermediate/long-acting insulin
Non-insulin dependent diabetes	Pre-pregnancy planning. Convert oral hypoglycaemic agents to human insulin pre-pregnancy
Gestational diabetes	Increase complex carbohydrate intake. Start human insulin if there is fasting or post prandial hyperglycaemia
Hypoglycaemia	Treat with milk. In serious situations give glucagon injection
Ketoacidosis	Correct metabolic acidosis conventionally. Treat underlying cause
Delivery	Give IV dextrose and potassium with insulin to maintain euglycaemia. Discontinue after delivery and restart pre-pregnancy insulin regime
Breastfeeding	Maintain metabolic control using an appropriate insulin regime

Thyroid disorders

Introduction

The management of thyroid disorders during pregnancy can be problematic as pregnancy may mimic the symptoms of thyroid disease. Thyroid function tests may also be altered, making diagnosis and management of the disease more difficult than in non-pregnant patients.

Alterations of thyroid hormones in pregnancy

Serum thyroxine binding globulin (TBG), total T_4 and T_3 gradually rise and may be above the normal range by the third trimester. Free T_4 and T_3 do not usually fluctuate greatly. Thyroid-stimulating hormone (TSH) may be below normal in the first trimester, but is usually normal in the third trimester. The most accurate assessment of thyroid function is therefore achieved by measuring free T_4 and T_3 and TSH levels.[16,17]

> **For the most accurate assessment of thyroid function, measure free T4, free T_3 and TSH levels.**

Hypothyroidism

This condition affects approximately ninc in 1000 pregnancies[18], although some publications suggest an incidence of approximately one in 2000 pregnancies.[19] Hypothyroidism is usually due to pre-existing thyroid autoimmune disease, previous thyroid surgery or radioactive iodine treatment. It occasionally occurs secondary to pituitary or hypothalamic disease, and rarely due to iodine deficiency or a congenital defect.[19]

Possible adverse maternal/fetal effects

Hypothyroidism may increase the risk of spontaneous abortion.[19,20] Uncontrolled hypothyroidism during pregnancy has been associated with premature labour, fetal loss, stillbirth, an increased risk of pre-eclampsia, abruptio placentae, anaemia and post-partum bleeding.[16] If untreated, the incidence of abnormalities has been reported to be as high as 11.6%, compared to 3% with controlled disease.[19]

> **Early diagnosis and good control of thyroid function during pregnancy improves maternal and fetal outcome.**

Diagnosis

Symptoms include weight gain, fatigue, cold intolerance, hair loss and dry skin. Free T_4 and T_3 levels may be normal or low, TSH levels are usually raised.[16,19]

Management

Treatment is with thyroxine replacement, with regular review of the dose due to increased requirements (50–100%) in pregnancy.[20,22] The aim is to keep the free T_4 level at the upper end of normal and the TSH in the normal range. The usual dose of thyroxine is 100 µg daily. If necessary the dose is increased by 25–50 µg every four weeks until symptomatic improvement occurs. Patients should be reviewed each trimester to ensure the free T_4 and TSH levels are in the required range. After delivery the thyroxine dose will need to be reduced to pre-pregnancy levels, and the free T_4 and TSH levels checked six to eight weeks later.[19]

Babies born to hypothyroid mothers should undergo a routine neonatal thyroid screen. Free T_4 and TSH levels should be taken from the cord blood due to thyroid-blocking antibodies crossing the placenta and possibly inducing neonatal hypothyroidism.[23]

> - **Regular review is needed as thyroxine requirements may increase.**
> - **Thyroxine doses need to be reduced after delivery.**
> - **A routine neonatal thyroid screen should be performed.**

Breastfeeding

Thyroxine treatment is not a contraindication to breastfeeding.[18]

Hyperthyroidism

Hyperthyroidism affects approximately two in 1000 pregnancies.[24] Ninety-five per cent of cases are due to pre-existing Graves' disease. Other causes are toxic solitary nodules, toxic multinodular goitre, Hashimoto's thyroiditis and trophoblastic disease.

Pre-existing hyperthyroidism may improve, especially in the latter half of pregnancy. However, previously controlled disease may relapse.[18]

Possible adverse maternal/fetal effects

Uncontrolled hyperthyroidism is associated with premature delivery, perinatal death, small-for-date babies and serious neonatal and maternal morbidity. The prognosis for the mother and baby depends on the time from onset to adequate control of the condition.[18,21] Congenital neonatal hyperthyroidism may occur as a result of thyroid antibody stimulation, or following inadvertent iodine use in early pregnancy.

> **Rapid control of thyroid function improves pregnancy outcome.**

Diagnosis

Accurate diagnosis of hyperthyroidism starting in pregnancy is difficult as the symptoms and signs are non-specific, e.g. heat intolerance, tachycardia and warm skin. Decreased weight, eye signs and thyroid bruit, along with the other symptoms and signs, are more suggestive. Raised free T_4 and T_3 levels confirm diagnosis, although in early disease only the T_3 may be raised.[24] TSH is suppressed and levels may be below the sensitivity of the test.

Scanning or radio-uptakes, e.g. ^{131}I or ^{99m}TC, should be avoided in pregnancy as the fetal thyroid is 20 to 50 times more avid for iodine than the maternal thyroid. If test or diagnostic doses are used inadvertently during early pregnancy, the amount of radioactive compound administered is unlikely to be harmful as the fetal thyroid is not fully functional until 10–12 weeks post-conception.[22,24]

- • **Accurate diagnosis is difficult.**
- • **Raised free T_4 and T_3 levels confirm diagnosis.**
- • **In early disease only the T_3 may be raised.**
- • **Avoid scanning or radio-uptakes, e.g. ^{131}I or ^{99m}TC.**

Management

Carbimazole, propylthiouracil (PTU) and, less commonly in the UK, methimazole, are the treatments of choice to control hyperthyroidism in pregnancy. They are equally effective, reducing thyroid levels to normal over a period of four to eight weeks.[22,24] There is a possible rare association between methimazole and congenital aplasia cutis, a localised skin defect usually occurring on the scalp.[25–27] PTU has a theoretical advantage over carbimazole as less crosses the placenta[28] and it partially inhibits the conversion of T_4 to T_3.[21] In practice, carbimazole is usually used due to greater experience with its use.

The doses of carbimazole and PTU should be the lowest possible that will maintain thyroid hormone levels in the upper normal range.[18,29] Over-treatment runs the risk of fetal goitre and hypothyroidism. Regular review, every four to six weeks, is necessary to maintain optimum control and thus minimise potential risk to the mother and fetus. If clinically possible, treatment should be reduced or discontinued three to four weeks before delivery to minimise the risk of neonatal complications.[16,24]

Block/replacement regimes, using higher than normal doses of carbimazole or PTU with a thyroxine supplement, are not recommended as little thyroxine crosses the placenta.[22] This may result in a euthyroid mother and a hypothyroid infant.[18,30]

Beta-blockers, such as propranolol, are only used for symptomatic relief in patients with severe hyperthyroidism while waiting for anti-thyroid treatment to take effect.[22,24]

Iodides should only be used for short-term treatment prior to surgery or in the event of thyrotoxic crisis ('thyroid storm'), and are therefore rarely necessary in pregnancy. They readily cross the placenta and may induce fetal hypothyroidism or goitres.[20]

Surgery in pregnancy is reserved for those patients not responding to, or intolerant of, anti-thyroid agents.

Radioactive iodine (^{131}I) is contra-indicated in pregnancy as it may permanently ablate the fetal thyroid gland.[31] A pregnancy test should be performed before treatment doses are used in a woman of child-bearing potential.

- Carbimazole and PTU are equally effective anti-thyroid drugs.
- Use the lowest possible dose to maintain thyroid hormone levels in the upper normal range.
- Review treatment every four to six weeks to maintain optimum control.
- Avoid block/replacement regimes and radioactive iodine.

Thyrotoxic crisis ('thyroid storm')

This is a medical emergency as there is considerable risk to both the mother and fetus. It may be precipitated by stress, such as infection, labour, Caesarean section or other surgery.[24] The fever associated with thyroid storm usually occurs within a few hours of the onset of the precipitating factor. Symptoms include tachycardia, restlessness, confusion, coma, nausea and vomiting. Intensive monitoring and treatment is required, and patients may need admission to an intensive treatment unit (ITU).

Breastfeeding

Carbimazole and PTU are both detectable in breast milk but the concentrations are thought to be insufficient to affect neonatal thyroid function.[32,33] Ideally, fetal thyroid function should be checked weekly for the first two weeks post-delivery.[34] If laboratory assessment is not possible, the infant should be examined for clinical signs of hypothyroidism and goitre.

Radioactive iodine (^{131}I) is contraindicated in breastfeeding. If a test dose is used a gap of 36 hours should be left between scanning and restarting feeding, whilst a diagnostic dose requires a gap of two weeks.[35] If a treatment dose is used, the levels excreted in breast milk are thought to be reduced to background levels after eight weeks.[31]

Summary

Adequate control of maternal hypo- and hyperthyroidism is the key to management and will minimise the potential risk to the fetus (Table 12.2).

Table 12.2: Management of maternal hypo- and hyperthyroidism

	Carbimazole	Propylthiouracil	Thyroxine
Usual doses	Treatment: 20–45 mg daily in divided doses	Treatment: 200–450 mg daily in three divided doses	Starting dose: 100 µg daily, adjusted as necessary
	Maintenance: 5–20 mg daily	Maintenance: 50–200 mg daily in three divided doses	Maintenance: 100–200 µg daily
Safety in pregnancy	Not thought to be associated with an increased risk of non-thyroid malformations	No evidence of increased fetal risk of non-thyroid malformations	No evidence of increased fetal risk of non-thyroid malformations
	Methimazole, a metabolite of carbimazole, has been linked with aplasia cutis although a causal relationship is unproven	Less PTU crosses the placenta in comparison with carbimazole	
Breastfeeding	May be used	May be used	May be used
		A lower concentration of PTU is present in breast milk in comparison with carbimazole	
Monitoring required – maternal	Free T_4, free T_3 and TSH + symptoms should be reviewed regularly	Free T_4, free T_3 and TSH + symptoms should be reviewed regularly	Free T_4, free T_3 and TSH + symptoms should be reviewed regularly
Monitoring required – fetal	Neonatal thyroid screen, including fetal heart rate, T_4 and TSH from cord blood	Neonatal thyroid screen, including fetal heart rate; T_4 and TSH from cord blood	Neonatal thyroid screen, T_4 and TSH from cord blood
	Repeat levels after three to seven days if taken up to delivery	Repeat levels after three to seven days if taken up to delivery	

References

1   Garner P (1995) Type I diabetes mellitus and pregnancy. *Lancet.* **346**: 157–61.

2   de Veciana M, Major CA, Morgan MA *et al.* (1995) Postprandial versus preprandial blood glucose monitoring in women with gestational diabetes mellitus requiring insulin treatment. *N Engl J Med.* **333**(19): 1237–41.

3   Kopelman P (1996) Gestational diabetes and beyond. *Lancet.* **347**: 208–9.

4   Casson IF, Clarke CA, Howard CV *et al.* (1997) Outcomes of pregnancy in insulin-dependent diabetic women: results of a five-year population cohort study. *BMJ.* **315**: 275–8.

5   Landon MB and Gabbe SG (1995) Diabetes mellitus. In *Medical Disorders During Pregnancy* (2nd edn) (eds WM Barron and MD Lindheimer). Mosby Year Books, St Louis.

6   Vaughan NJA (1995) Treatment of diabetes. In *Prescribing in Pregnancy* (2nd edn) (ed P Rubin). BMJ Publishing Group, London.

7   Littley MD (1994) Management of diabetic pregnancy. *Postgrad Med J.* **70**: 610–19.

8   Kitzmiller JL, Buchanan TA, Kjos S *et al.* (1996) Pre-conception care of diabetes, congenital malformations and spontaneous abortions. *Diabet Care.* **19**(5): 514–41.

9   From Teratogen Information System (TERIS). 1974–1996 Micromedex Inc. Vol. 99.

10 Reece EA and Homko CJ (1998) Diabetes mellitus in pregnancy. What are the best treatment options? *Drug Safety.* **18**: 209–20.

11 Reece EA, Homko CJ and Wiznitzer A (1994) Hypoglycaemia in pregnancies complicated by diabetes mellitus: maternal and fetal considerations. *Clin Obstet Gynecol.* **37**: 50–8.

12 Steel JM and Johnstone FD (1996) Guidelines for the management of insulin-dependent diabetes mellitus in pregnancy. *Drugs.* **52**(1): 60–70.

13 Hagay ZJ (1994) Diabetic ketoacidosis in pregnancy: etiology, pathophysiology and management. *Clin Obstet Gynecol.* **37**(1): 39–49.

14 Briggs GG, Freeman RK and Yaffe SJ (1994) *Drugs in Pregnancy and Lactation* (4th edn). Williams & Wilkins, Baltimore.

15 Dollery C (1991) *Therapeutic Drugs.* Churchill Livingstone, Edinburgh.

16 (1995) The practical management of thyroid disease in pregnancy. *Drug Ther Bull.* **33**: 75–7.

17 Brent GA (1997) Maternal thyroid function: interpretation of thyroid function tests in pregnancy. *Clin Obstet Gynecol.* **40**(1): 3–15.

18 Girling JC (1996) Thyroid disease and pregnancy. *Br J Hosp Med.* **56**(7): 316–20.

19 Montoro MN (1997) Management of hypothyroidism during pregnancy. *Clin Obstet Gynecol.* **40**(1): 65–80.

20 Mazzaferri EL (1997) Evaluation and management of common thyroid disorders in women. *Am J Obstet Gynecol.* **176**: 507–14.

21 Giardina S, Contrarini A and Becca B (1993) Maternal diseases and congenital malformations. *Ann Ist Super.* **29**: 69–76.

22 Roti E, Minelli R and Salvi M (1996) Management of hyperthyroidism and hypothyroidism in the pregnant woman. *J Clin Endocrinol Metab.* **81**(5): 1679–82.

23 Ramsay I (1995) Thyroid disease. In *Medical Disorders in Obstetric Practice* (3rd edn) (ed M de Swiet). Blackwell Science, Oxford.

24 Mestman JH (1997) Hyperthyroidism in pregnancy. *Clin Obstet Gynecol.* **40**(1): 45–64.

25 Mandel SJ, Brent GA and Larsen PR (1994) Review of anti-thyroid drug use during pregnancy and report of a case of aplasia cutis. *Thyroid.* **4**: 129–33.

26 Wing DA, Millar LK, Koonings PP *et al.* (1994) A comparison of propylthiouracil versus methimazole in the treatment of hyperthyroidism in pregnancy. *Am J Obstet Gynecol.* **170**: 90–5.

27 Thomas CL (ed) (1993) *Taber's Cyclopedic Medical Dictionary* (17th edn). FA Davis Company, Philadelphia.

28 Rosen H (1986) Treatment of thyrotoxicosis in pregnancy. *N Engl J Med.* **314**: 849.

29 Belchetz PE (1987) Thyroid disease in pregnancy. *BMJ.* **294**: 264–5.

30 Hall R, Richards CJ and Lazarus JH (1993) The thyroid and pregnancy. *Br J Obstet Gynecol.* **100**: 512–15.

31 Anon (1993) Radio-iodine for the treatment of thyroid disease. *Drug Ther Bull.* **31**: 39–40.

32 Cooper DS (1987) Antithyroid drugs: to breast-feed or not to breast-feed. *Am J Obstet Gynecol.* **157**: 234–5.

33 Momotani N, Yamashiti R, Yoshimoto M *et al.* (1989) Recovery from fetal hypothyroidism: evidence for the safety of breastfeeding while taking propylthiouracil. *Clin Endocrinol.* **31**: 591–5.

34 Lamberg BA, Ikonen E, Osterlund K *et al.* (1984) Anti-thyroid treatment of maternal hyperthyroidism during lacatation. *Clin Endocrinol.* **21**: 81–7.

35 Lawrence RA (1994) *Breastfeeding: a guide for the medical professional* (4th edn). Mosby Year Books, St Louis.

CHAPTER THIRTEEN

Nutrition in pregnancy

Martin Parkinson

Diet

Dietary advice in preparation for, and during, pregnancy is aimed at reducing both the risks of birth defects and of having an infant of low birth weight that is at increased risk of poor health. There is, however, controversy about the relationship between the mother's diet and fetal well-being. Observational studies in this area have yielded conflicting results, mainly because so many aspects of the pregnant woman's life vary with diet and nutrition. Adequate controlled studies have been too small to allow firm conclusions to be drawn.[1]

Dietary restriction in pregnancy causes decreased birth weight but it is not clear whether this is associated with an effect on morbidity and mortality. Nutritional protein supplements may lead to a modest increase in birth weight but no other benefits are recognised. There is no evidence that any kind of dietary modification will help prevent pre-eclampsia. Women should not be told to restrict their diet to avoid 'high' weight gain. There is no evidence that reducing salt intake is helpful; one study found a lower incidence of pre-eclampsia in women advised to eat more salt than in those advised to eat less.[2] There is no evidence that dietary restriction of any sort is beneficial to pregnant women or their babies. Observational studies have reported that gestational weight gain is positively correlated with fetal growth and possibly with a reduced risk of pre-term birth. In addition, there is some evidence that energy/protein restriction is associated with impaired fetal growth.

Most studies that have attempted to determine the benefits of nutritional supplements on gestational weight gain and pregnancy outcome have serious flaws in the methodology.[3–7] Energy supplements appeared to be associated with enhanced fetal growth. Postnatal follow up has only been addressed in a few trials and in these there was no evidence of a lasting size advantage or improved cognitive development. There was no evidence of a reduction in stillbirth or neonatal death.

Women should be advised to maintain a healthy, balanced diet throughout pregnancy which includes sufficient iron and folate (Box 13.1).

Box 13.1:   Dietary advice for pregnancy and preconceptual care

- Eat plenty of foods rich in iron.
- Eat plenty of foods rich in folates (green leafy vegetables, e.g. spinach, cabbage, brussel sprouts, broccoli; breakfast cereals which are fortified with folic acid).
- Take a folic acid supplement (400 µg daily) from planning to conceive until 12 weeks pregnant (higher dose necessary if previous child with neural tube defect or taking anti-epileptics).
- Avoid liver or liver products (pâtés, etc) (*see* 'Vitamin A', p. 170).
- Do not take vitamin A supplements other than on medical advice.
- Avoid foods associated with risk of listeriosis (*see* Chapter 11).
- Avoid alcohol (*see* Chapter 17).
- Vegetarians/vegans should also take an oral vitamin B_{12} supplement.
- Unless a woman has malnutrition or a known deficiency state there is no need to take supplements other than folic acid.

Folic acid and the prevention of neural tube defects

Folic acid is a group B vitamin. Its active metabolites (mainly folinic acid) act as coenzymes in many biochemical pathways, particularly purine and pyrimidine synthesis, and amino acid metabolism. Folic acid has an indirect action on rapidly dividing tissues (e.g. blood stem cells, epithelial cells and fetal tissues). After the discovery that aminopterin, a folic acid antagonist, could cause birth defects, a number of studies examined the possible link between maternal blood folate levels in early pregnancy and the risk of fetal malformations, with contradictory results.[8–10] Studies were then carried out to identify whether peri-conceptual folate or multivitamins would prevent neural tube defects (NTDs) in women who had previously given birth to an affected child.[11–13]

During fetal development, the formation and closure of the neural tube occurs in two stages, primary and secondary neurulation. In primary neurulation, the neural plate ectoderm undergoes folding which leads to the formation of a closed tube. This process is responsible for the formation of the brain and part of the spinal cord, and occurs between the third and fourth weeks of gestation. Secondary neurulation occurs by a different process; it is mainly abnormalities of primary neurulation which result in neural tube defects.

Neural tube defects are divided into three types; anencephaly, encephalocoele and spina bifida. The prevalence of NTDs at birth in the UK population is now less than 0.3 per 1000 total births. However, the risk of recurrence is high, i.e. a woman who has previously had an affected child has a risk 10 times greater than that in the general population.[14]

There is good evidence that women who boost their intake of folic acid are less likely to have a child with a NTD.[15,16] Deficiency of folic acid might contribute to NTDs; mothers of affected children appear to handle folic acid abnormally. However, the cause of NTDs is likely to be multifactorial and not all can be prevented by folic acid supplements.

Primary prevention of neural tube defects (Boxes 13.2 to 13.4)

Epidemiological case–control and cohort studies favour a protective effect of folic acid supplementation in women with no relevant history.[13,17] A study involving more than 5000 women found that almost 60% fewer pregnancies were associated with a first occurrence of NTDs following administration of a multivitamin supplement, including 800 microgrammes of folic acid, than in those given a similar preparation without folic acid.[13] No protection was observed in women who started folic acid after the seventh week of gestation.[18]

Based on the results of these and other studies, the Department of Health recommends that all women wishing to become pregnant should take a folic acid supplement of 400 microgrammes daily from when they plan to have a baby until the 12th week of pregnancy. The available evidence is inadequate to assess the magnitude of the effect, nor does it allow firm conclusions about what dose is most effective. Preparations containing 400 microgrammes of folic acid may be prescribed or bought from community pharmacies. In the UK, whether bread should be fortified with folate is currently under discussion.

Box 13.2:   Preventing first occurrence of a neural tube defect

All women planning a pregnancy should take 400 microgrammes folic acid daily before conception and until the 12th week of gestation.

Neural tube defect recurrence

Several studies have shown that folic acid supplementation (0.36 mg–5 mg) starting one month before conception and continued until the end of the third month of pregnancy reduces the risk of NTD in the offspring of women with a positive history.[19] A randomised double-blind trial involving 1817 such women showed that folic acid 4 mg daily from before conception until the 12th week of pregnancy decreased NTD recurrence by 72%.[20] Folic acid tablets 5 mg are available only on prescription; as yet there is no licensed preparation in the UK containing 4 mg.

Box 13.3: Prevention of neural tube defect recurrence

- Folic acid supplements taken from before conception until the 12th week of pregnancy significantly decrease the risk of NTD recurrence.
- All women who have had a pregnancy affected by a NTD should receive folic acid 4 or 5 mg daily from before conception until the 12th week of pregnancy.

Women taking anti-epileptics

It is difficult to assess the influence of folates on the risk of congenital malformations in women with epilepsy (*see* Chapter 9). All anti-epileptic drugs have been implicated in congenital malformations, especially cleft palate and heart defects. Women on sodium valproate[21] or carbamazepine[22] therapy are at increased risk of having a baby with a NTD. The role of folate in anti-epileptic teratogenicity is still unclear.[23,24] It has been shown that women with epilepsy who had abnormal pregnancy outcomes had significantly lower blood folate concentrations.[25] However, phenytoin and barbiturates, the anti-epileptic drugs with most effect on folic acid status, pose the lowest risk for fetal NTDs. Conversely, sodium valproate and carbamazepine have less effect on folic acid.[14]

Few studies have assessed the influence of folic acid supplementation on pregnancy outcome in women with epilepsy. The rate of birth defects was determined in a prospective follow-up study of 33 neonates whose mothers had received 2.5–5 mg daily of folic acid during the pregnancy (starting before conception in 26 cases). There were no malformations but the study was too small to draw firm conclusions.[26] Although firm evidence that folic acid supplementation has a protective effect is lacking, such an effect seems likely.[27]

Most experts recommend that women taking any anti-epileptic drug should take a 5 mg daily dose of folic acid whether or not they have had an affected baby.[28,29] Taking folic acid should not discourage women from undergoing screening for NTDs. Concern that folic acid supplementation may interfere with the efficacy of some anti-epileptics, leading to a deterioration in seizure control, is unfounded.[28,30] Three randomised controlled trials involving about 150 women with epilepsy showed that supplementation for three months to a year (10–15 mg daily) did not alter seizure control.[31–33]

Box 13.4: Prevention of neural tube defects in women on anti-epileptics

- Carbamazepine and sodium valproate exposure during pregnancy increase the risk of NTDs.
- Women on any anti-epileptic drug should take a folic acid supplement of 5 mg daily from before conception until the 12th week of gestation.

Iron

The UK diet contains up to 20 mg iron daily. During pregnancy the iron requirement increases threefold to about 6 mg daily; extra is needed for the increase in maternal red cells and for fetal and placental development.[34,35] Iron absorption is increased in pregnancy and there is a saving of the iron normally lost through menstruation.[36,37] The average net iron loss to the mother, which occurs mainly in the second and third trimesters, is around 600 mg. To meet this the mother needs an additional 2 mg of iron daily. During pregnancy the proportion of ingested iron absorbed varies from 10% to 90%.

Some women are unable to meet the increased demand without depleting their iron stores and, as a result, may become anaemic. Between the late 1950s and 1980s it was common practice to give supplements to all pregnant women. More recently this has been criticised and debated, and the controversy is not yet resolved.[36,37]

Low haemoglobin concentrations are a normal physiologic response to the plasma volume expansion that occurs in pregnancy. The normal pattern is for haemoglobin concentrations to fall to a nadir in the second trimester and rise thereafter, approaching pre-pregnancy levels by term.[38,39] Mean cell volume is unaffected by pregnancy and offers a better measure of iron-deficiency anaemia.[40]

Correction of anaemia (Box 13.5)

Studies in the United States and Europe have suggested that even mild to moderate anaemia can be associated with adverse pregnancy outcome, including low birth weight, pre-term birth and perinatal death.[36–39] However, it is unclear whether anaemia is responsible for these outcomes and whether they can be prevented through iron supplementation.

Iron treatment of a low haemoglobin, without other evidence of iron deficiency, is seldom necessary. Supplementation clearly changes the blood picture towards its non-pregnant state, but this has not been shown to confer any benefit on either mother or baby. Indeed, treatment may be harmful. Two well-conducted trials found that iron supplements resulted in an increase in the prevalence of pre-term delivery and low birth weight.[40] It has been postulated that iron-induced macrocytosis and increased haemoglobin concentration may increase the viscosity of maternal blood and thus impede uteroplacental blood flow.

Iron therapy should be given if there is evidence of deficiency.

Box 13.5:   Correction of anaemia

- Iron supplements should be given if there is evidence of iron deficiency anaemia in the first trimester.
- Later in pregnancy, iron supplements should be considered if the haemoglobin concentration falls below 10 g/dL or the mean cell volume below 82 fl.
- With supplementation, the haemoglobin can be expected to increase at a rate of 0.8 g/dL per week.
- Parenteral iron may be required if deficiency is recognised late in pregnancy.
- Transfusion may be indicated if there is not time to achieve a satisfactory response before delivery.

Routine vs selective supplementation (Box 13.6)

Controlled trials evaluating routine iron supplementation (of about 100 mg elemental iron daily) show that it raises or maintains the serum ferritin above 10 microgrammes/L, resulting in a substantial reduction in the proportion of women with a haemoglobin level below 10 g/dL in late pregnancy.

However, routine supplementation in well-nourished women has no detectable effect on any substantial measures of either maternal or fetal outcome. Hemminki and Starfield[41] reviewed controlled clinical trials of iron administration during pregnancy in developed Western countries. They concluded that there was no beneficial effect in terms of birth weight and maternal and infant morbidity and mortality, in those women receiving iron compared with controls. The only possible advantage was a reduced likelihood of Caesarean section and post-partum blood transfusion. The same investigators reported long-term follow-up (seven years) in 2682 women and their infants who had taken part in a study comparing routine iron prophylaxis with as-required therapy.[42] The only statistically significant difference was that infants of the routinely supplemented group were more frequently hospitalised because of convulsions.

The argument for more widespread supplementation centres on the observation that a high proportion of women in their reproductive years lack storage iron.[43,44] It has been suggested that women at risk of iron-deficiency anaemia could be identified by estimating the serum ferritin concentration in the first trimester. A value of less than 50 microgrammes/L in early pregnancy would be an indication for supplementation. Women with a serum ferritin concentration greater than 80 microgrammes/L are unlikely to require supplements.[45] Available data suggest that as many as 80% of women in the UK would be eligible for supplementation by these criteria.

The Cochrane Library review on this issue concludes that there is no evidence to advise against a policy of routine iron supplementation in pregnancy.[46] Routine supplementation could be warranted in populations in which iron deficiency is common.[46] Supplements are advisable in women at greater risk of anaemia including those who have had menorrhagia, or repeated closely spaced pregnancies or miscarriage, and those with a poor diet.

Choice of preparation

Ferrous sulphate is as effective and less expensive than other products and is the drug of choice. Adverse gastrointestinal effects are common with standard doses and include metallic taste, heartburn, nausea and constipation. Although modified-release products are claimed to have fewer gastrointestinal effects, they are poorly absorbed and should not be used. Preparations containing ascorbic acid or chelated iron to facilitate absorption offer no therapeutic advantage.

This hypothesis that weekly iron administration may be as effective as daily dosing is supported by animal studies but few trials have investigated this in humans.[47] In a study in 139 pregnant women, comparable effects on haemoglobin and serum ferritin were achieved with a weekly dose of 120 mg ferrous sulphate and a daily dose of 60 mg.[48] This approach requires further study.

Box 13.6:   Iron supplementation

- Routine iron supplementation does not effect maternal or fetal morbidity.
- Iron supplements should be administered to women who have significant anaemia or are at increased risk of anaemia.
- Ferrous sulphate is the drug of choice; other iron formulation preparations and sustained-release dosage forms offer no advantages.

Vitamins

Vitamin A (Box 13.7)

Vitamin A is required for normal vision, reproduction, maintenance of epithelial tissue and for growth and bone development. The term vitamin A refers to retinoid compounds that have the biological activity of retinol. Retinol is a fat-soluble essential vitamin which occurs naturally in a variety of foods such as dairy products and liver. Beta-carotene and other carotenoids are plant-synthesised precursors of vitamin A that are partially converted to retinol during or after absorption. Retinoids are known teratogens in animals, both high and low levels may result in fetal malformations.[49,50] In humans, isotretinoin, the synthetic retinoid used in acne treatment, causes congenital abnormalities. [51]

Cases suggesting a link between excessive vitamin A ingestion during pregnancy and fetal malformations have been reported.[52] In 1987, women in the USA were recommended not to take more than 10 000 IU of vitamin A per day.[53] Since then two case–control studies have concluded that children born to women consuming vitamin A at levels found in supplements are not at increased risk for birth defects.[54,55] A recent prospective study[56] investigating birth defects and the intake of vitamin A from food and supplements in almost 23 000 pregnant women found that consumption of less than 10 000 IU of vitamin A appeared safe. However, the authors estimated that the ingestion of larger amounts was associated with birth defects in one in 57 babies. There was a marked increase in incidence of birth defects of structures arising from the cranial neural crest (craniofacial, central nervous system, thymic and heart defects). These data indicate that large doses of vitamin A must be regarded as potentially harmful to the fetus.

Severe maternal vitamin A deficiency has been asociated with a variety of fetal abnormalities mainly affecting the eyes; such deficiency is rare.

The average balanced daily diet contains approximately 7000–8000 IU of vitamin A. Doses in excess of the UK reference nutrient intake (RNI) (about 5000 IU/day) should be avoided by women who are, or may become, pregnant. Women who are, or may become, pregnant should be advised not to take vitamin A supplements (including fish-liver oil). They should avoid eating liver or liver products. Vitamin A supplements should only be prescribed when there is clear evidence of deficiency.

Box 13.7:   Vitamin A

- Excessive doses during pregnancy may result in birth defects.
- Daily doses of 15 000 IU or more are potentially harmful.
- Women who are, or wish to become, pregnant should not routinely take vitamin A supplements, nor should they eat liver or liver-based products.

Vitamin C (Box 13.8)

Vitamin C (ascorbic acid) is a water-soluble essential nutrient required for collagen formation, tissue repair, conversion of folic to folinic acid, and iron metabolism together with several other metabolic processes. Deficiency is associated with scurvy. The UK RNI for women aged 19 to 50 years is 600 mg.

Maternal vitamin C levels decline slowly during pregnancy, and the mother may develop an asymptomatic deficiency state. However, studies have found no association between deficiency and either maternal or fetal complications, including congenital abnormalities.[57] There is no evidence that excessive doses of vitamin C are harmful to the mother or fetus. Vitamin C supplements may be given where the diet is poor.

Box 13.8:   Vitamin C

- Excessive doses do not appear to cause harm to the fetus.
- Pregnant women should take an additional 10 mg over the RNI.

Vitamin D (Box 13.9)

Vitamin D analogues are fat-soluble vitamins with anti-rachitic and hypercalcaemic activity. The two naturally biologically active forms of vitamin D are produced by the action of ultraviolet light on vitamin D provitamins.

High doses of vitamin D are teratogenic in animals but there is no conclusive evidence of problems in humans. Due to its effects on calcium metabolism, the role of vitamin D has been questioned in the pathogenesis of supravalvular aortic stenosis syndrome, which is often associated with hypercalcaemia of infancy.[58–60] This extremely rare syndrome comprises mental and growth retardation and supravalvular aortic and pulmonary stenosis. However, excessive maternal intake or retention of vitamin D has not been consistently found in affected infants. The very high-dose levels (daily doses averaging 107 000 IU) of vitamin D used to treat maternal hypoparathyroidism during pregnancy have not been associated with fetal abnormalities.[61]

Severe vitamin D deficiency during pregnancy may lead to maternal and fetal adverse effects. Osteomalacia may lead to decreased weight gain and pelvic deformities which may interfere with normal vaginal delivery.[62] Possible adverse effects on the fetus include hypocalcaemia and neonatal rickets.

Box 13.9:   Vitamin D

- Deficiency during pregnancy has been linked with maternal and fetal adverse effects.
- There is no evidence that excessive vitamin D intake has adverse effects on the fetus.
- Supplements may be given if required.

Vitamin E (Box 13.10)

Vitamin E and its analogues are essential for normal health, although their biological function is unclear. Deficiency is uncommon during pregnancy but no maternal or fetal abnormalities have been identified.[57]

Vitamin E has been investigated in the prevention of abortion and premature labour but there was no evidence of efficacy. Supplements have also been given in an attempt to prevent neonatal complications of inadequate vitamin E intake in the first month after birth. Doses in excess of the RNI have not proved to be harmful.

Box 13.10:   Vitamin E

- Deficiency is uncommon, and is not associated with fetal or maternal harm.
- Doses in excess of the RNI have not been associated with fetal harm.

Multivitamin preparations

Vitamin and mineral supplementation during pregnancy is common, in one study conducted in the United States, 23% of women questioned during antenatal clinics were taking some form of vitamin supplement during pregnancy.[63] Factors which affected supplementation included advice received from diverse sources and whether or not the women were also taking iron supplements. However, supplementation did not appear to be affected by age, social class or reproductive history. Despite the relatively common practice, multivitamin supplementation is rarely necessary during pregnancy. A study carried out by the Nutrition Unit of the World Health Organisation found no effect of vitamin supplementation on the occurrence of intrauterine growth retardation.[64] It is important that women do not assume that taking a multivitamin negates the need for folic acid, as the quantity of folic acid in many multivitamin preparations is less than that required in pregnancy.

Zinc and trace elements

Zinc deficiency is relatively common, especially in areas where the population subsists on cereal proteins. Zinc deficiency in pregnancy is associated with increased maternal morbidity, prolonged gestation or pre-term delivery and increased fetal risk. There is no need to routinely screen pregnant women for trace-element status. The best indicators that a woman's trace-element status may be sub-optimal are a history of poor food selection, a clinical disorder that alters trace-element use or excretion, or residence in an area with low trace-element content in soil. Routine supplementation in pregnancy is not recommended.[65,66]

References

1   *The Cochrane Library* (1999) Update Software, Oxford.
2   Anon (1995) Dietary modification in pregnancy. In *A Guide to Effective Care in Pregnancy and Childbirth* (2nd ed) (eds M Enkin, MJNC Keirse, M Renfrew *et al.*) Oxford University Press, Oxford.
3   Blackwell RQ, Chow BF, Chinn KSK *et al.* (1973) Prospective maternal nutrition study in Taiwan: rationale, study design, feasibility and preliminary findings. *Nutr Rep Int.* **7**: 517–32.
4   Elwood PC, Haley TJL, Sweetham PM *et al.* (1981) Child growth 0–5 years and the effect of entitlement to a milk supplement. *Arch Dis Child.* **56**: 831–5.
5   Kardjati S, Kusin JA and de With C (1989) Energy supplementation in the last trimester of pregnancy in East Java. 1. Effect on birth weight. *Br J Obstet Gynaecol.* **95**: 783–94.

6   Mora JO, Clement J, Christiansen N *et al.* (1978) Nutritional supplementation and the outcome of pregnancy. III Perinatal and neonatal mortality. *Nutr Rep Int.* **18**: 167–75.

7   Rush D, Stein Z and Susser M (1980) A randomised controlled trial of perinatal nutritional supplementation in New York City. *Pediatrics.* **65**: 683–97.

8   Hibbard ED and Smithells WN (1965) Folic acid metabolism and human embryopathy. *Lancet.* **i**: 1254–5.

9   Hall MH (1972) Folic acid deficiency and congenital malformation. *J Obstet Gynecol Br Commonwealth.* **79**: 159–61.

10   Hibbard BM (1975) Folates and the fetus. *S Afr Med J.* **49**: 1223–6.

11   Smithells RW, Nevin NC, Seller MJ *et al.* (1983) Further experience of vitamin supplementation for prevention of neural tube defect recurrences. *Lancet.* **i**: 1027–31.

12   Laurence KM, James N, Miller MH *et al.* (1981) Double-blind randomised controlled trial of folate treatment before conception to prevent recurrence of neural tube defects. *BMJ.* **282**: 1509–11.

13   Mulinare J, Cordero JF, Erickson JD *et al.* (1988) Periconceptual use of multivitamins and the occurrence of neural tube defects. *JAMA.* **260**: 3141–5.

14   Lewis DP, van Dyke DC, Stumbo P *et al.* (1998) Drug and environmental factors associated with adverse pregnancy outcomes. Part I: Anti-epileptic drugs, contraceptives, smoking and folate. *Ann Pharmacother.* **32**: 802–17.

15   MRC Vitamin Study Research Group (1991) Prevention of neural tube defects: results of the Medical Research Council Vitamin Study. *Lancet.* **346**: 393–6.

16   Czeizel AE and Dudas I (1992) Prevention of the first occurrence of neural tube defects by periconceptual vitamin supplementation. *N Engl J Med.* **327**: 1832–5.

17   Milunsky A, Jick H, Jick SS *et al.* (1989) Multivitamin folic acid supplementation in early pregnancy reduces the prevalence of neural tube defects. *JAMA.* **262**: 2847–52.

18   Czeizel A, Dudas I, Metneki J *et al.* (1994) Pregnancy outcomes in a randomised controlled trial of periconceptual multivitamin supplentation. *Arch Gynecol Obstet.* **255**: 131–9.

19   Anon (1996) Pregnancy: folic acid and prevention of neural tube defects. *Prescrib Int.* **5**: 53–7.

20   MRC Vitamin Study Research Group (1991) Prevention of neural tube defects: results of the Medical Research Council Vitamin Study. *Lancet.* **338**: 131–7.

21   Robert E and Guibaud P (1982) Maternal valproic acid and congenital neural tube defects. *Lancet.* **11**: 937.

22   Rosa FW (1991) Spina bifida in infants of women treated with carbamazepine during pregnancy. *N Engl J Med.* **324**: 674–7.

23   Lewis DP, van Dyke DC, Willhite LA *et al.* (1995) Phenytoin-folic acid interaction. *Ann Pharmacother.* **29**: 726–35.

24   van Dyke DC, Berg MJ and Olson CH (1991) Differences in phenytoin biotransformation and susceptibility to congenital malformations: a review. DICP *Ann Pharmacother.* **25**: 987–92.

25   Dansky LV, Rosenblat DS and Andermann E (1992) Mechanisms of teratogenesis: folic acid and anti-epileptic drug therapy. *Neurology.* **42**: 32–42.

26   Biale Y and Lewenthal H (1984) Effect of folic acid supplementation on congenital malformations due to anticonvulsive drugs. *Eur J Obstet Gyne Reprod Biol.* **18**: 211–16.

27   Dansky LV, Andermann E, Rosenblatt D *et al.* (1987) Anticonvulsants, folate levels, and pregnancy outcome: a prospective study. *Ann Neurol.* **21**: 176–82.

28 Cleland PG (1996) Management of pre-existing disorders in pregnancy: epilepsy. *Prescrib J.* **36**(2): 102–9.

29 Anon (1994) Epilepsy and pregnancy. *Drug Ther Bull.* **7**: 49–51.

30 Lindhout D and Omtzigt JGC (1994) Teratogenic effects of anti-epileptic drugs: implications for the management of epilepsy in women of child-bearing age. *Epilepsia.* **35**(4)S19–S28.

31 Gibberd FB, Nicholls A, Wright MG *et al.* (1981) The influence of folic acid on the frequency of epileptic attacks. *Eur J Clin Pharmacol.* **19**: 57–60.

32 Norris JW and Pratt RF (1971) A controlled study of folic acid in epilepsy. *Neurology.* **21**: 659–64.

33 Mattson RH, Gallagher BB, Reynolds EH *et al.* (1993) Folate therapy in epilepsy. A controlled study. *Arch Neurol.* **29**: 78–81.

34 Hytten FE and Leitch I (1971) The volume and composition of the blood. In *The Physiology of Human Pregnancy* (2nd edn), pp. 1–68. Blackwell Scientific, Oxford.

35 Barrett JFR, Whittaker PG, Williams JG *et al.* (1994) Absorption of non-haem iron from food during normal pregnancy. *BMJ.* **309**: 79–82.

36 Anon (1994) Routine iron supplements in pregnancy are unnecessary. *Drug Ther Bull.* **32**(4): 30–1.

37 United States Preventive Services Task Force (1993) Routine iron supplementation during pregnancy. *JAMA.* **270**: 2848–54.

38 Garn SM, Ridela SA, Petzoid AS *et al.* (1981) Maternal hematologic levels and pregnancy outcome. *Semin Perinatol.* **5**: 155–62.

39 Lieberman E, Ryan KJ, Monson RR *et al.* (1991) Association of maternal hematocrit with premature labor. *Am J Obstet Gynecol.* **164**: 59–63.

40 Klebanoff MA, Shiono PH, Selby JV *et al.* (1991) Anaemia and spontaneous pre-term birth. *Am J Obstet Gynecol.* **164**: 59–63.

41 Hemminki E and Starfield B (1978) Routine administration of iron and vitamins during pregnancy: review of controlled clinical trials. *Br J Obstet Gynecol.* **85**: 404–10.

42 Hemminki E and Merilainen J (1995) Long-term follow-up of mothers and their infants in a randomised trial on iron prophylaxis during pregnancy. *Am J Obstet Gynecol.* **173**: 205–9.

43 Fenton V, Cavill I and Fisher J (1977) Iron stores in pregnancy. *Br J Haematol.* **37**: 145–9.

44 de Leeuw NKM, Lowenstein L and Hsieh YS (1966) Iron deficiency and hydremia in normal pregnancy. *Medicine (Baltimore).* **45**: 291–315.

45 Letsky E (1995) Blood volume, haematinics, anaemia. In *Medical Disorders in Obstetric Practice* (3rd edn) (ed M de Swiet). Blackwell Scientific, Oxford.

46 Mahomed K (1999) *Iron supplementation in pregnancy.* (Cochrane Review). *The Cochrane Library*, Issue 3. Update Software, Oxford.

47 Viteri FE (1996) Weekly compared with daily iron supplementation. *Am J Clin Nutr.* **63**: 610.

48 Ridwan E, Schutlink W, Dillon D *et al.* (1996) Effects of weekly iron supplementation on pregnant Indonesian women are similar to those of daily supplementation. *Am J Clin Nutr.* **63**: 884–90.

49 Cohlan SQ (1954) Congenital anomalies in the rat produced by excessive intake of vitamin A during pregnancy. *Pediatrics.* **13**: 556–7.

50 Pinnock CB and Alderman CP (1992) The potential for teratogenicity of vitamin A and its cogeners. *Med J Aust.* **157**: 804–9.

51 Rosa FW (1983) Teratogenicity of isotretinoin. *Lancet.* **2**: 513.

52 Rosa FW, Wilk AL and Kelsey FO (1986) Teratogen update: vitamin A congeners. *Teratology.* **33**: 355–64.

53 Centers for Disease Control, US Dept of Health and Human Services (1987) Use of supplements containing high-dose vitamin A – New York State 1983–84. *MMWR.* **36**: 80–2.

54 Martinez-Frias ML and Salvador J (1990) Epidemiological aspects of prenatal exposure to high doses of vitamin A in Spain. *Eur J Epidemiol.* **6**: 118–23.

55 Werler MM, Lammer EJ, Rosenberg L *et al.* (1990) Maternal vitamin A supplementation in relation to selected birth defects. *Teratology.* **42**: 497–503.

56 Rothman KJ, Moore LL, Singer MR *et al.* (1995) Teratogenicity of high vitamin A intake. *New Engl J Med.* **333**: 1369–73.

57 Briggs GG, Freeman RK and Yaffe SJ (1994) *Drugs in Pregnancy and Lactation. A reference guide to fetal and neonatal risk* (4th edn). Williams and Wilkins, Baltimore.

58 Friedman WF and Mills L (1969). The relationship between vitamin D and the craniofacial and dental anomalies of supravalvular aortic stenosis syndrome. *Pediatrics.* **43**: 12–18.

59 Rowe RD and Cooke RE (1969) Vitamin D and craniofacial and dental anomalies of supravalvular stenosis syndrome. *Pediatrics.* **43**: 1–2.

60 Taussig HB (1966) Possible injury to the cardiovascular system from vitamin D. *Ann Intern Med.* **65**: 1195–200.

61 Goodenday LS and Gordon GS (1971) No risk from vitamin D in pregnancy. *Ann Intern Med.* **75**: 807–8.

62 Pitkin RM (1985) Calcium metabolism in pregnancy and the perinatal period: a review. *Am J Obstet Gynecol.* **151**: 99–109.

63 Best A, Little J and MacPherson M (1989) Vitamin supplementation in pregnancy. *J R Soc Hlth.* **109**(2): 60–3.

64 De Onis M, Villar J and Gulmezoglu M (1998) Nutritional interventions to prevent intrauterine growth retardation: evidence from randomised controlled trials. *Eur J Clin Nutr.* **52**(1): S83–S93.

65 Prasad AS (1996) Zinc deficiency in women, infants and children. *J Am Coll Nutr.* **15**(2): 113–20.

66 Wada L and King JC (1994) Trace-element nutrition during pregnancy. *Clin Obstet Gynecol.* **37**(3): 574–86.

CHAPTER FOURTEEN

Rheumatic disorders

Phil Young

Introduction

> - **Rheumatoid arthritis and systemic lupus erythematosus are the most frequently encountered rheumatic disorders in pregnancy.**
> - **Symptoms of rheumatic disorders often improve in pregnancy without treatment.**

Rheumatic disease is characterised by inflammation, with the joints, skin and kidney most frequently involved. They are more common in women, and several, including rheumatoid arthritis and systemic lupus erythematosus (SLE), occur preferentially in women of child-bearing age.[1,2]

Active rheumatic disease during pregnancy may require drug treatment to ensure the mother's health is maintained and that there is good fetal outcome. As the data on pregnancy outcome after exposure to anti-rheumatic drugs are limited, decision making can be difficult for both patient and physician. The activity of the disorder at the time of pregnancy and possible effects on the fetus must also be considered. Rheumatoid arthritis may cause reduced fertility in women,[3,4] although this requires confirmation.

Rheumatoid arthritis

> - **During pregnancy symptoms improve in about 75% of women and worsen in 5%.**
> - **The disease course during any previous pregnancy is predictive of the course in subsequent pregnancies.**

Rheumatoid arthritis (RA) has a prevalence of about 2–3%. It is three times more common in women with a peak prevalence in women aged 20–40 years.[1] The condition may develop for the first time during pregnancy, usually in the second or third trimester.[5] In about three-quarters of pregnant women symptoms improve, often in the first trimester, but in some not until later.[6,7] In about 5% of women symptoms worsen and new joint lesions develop.

Few prospective studies have evaluated the effects of RA on pregnancy.[7–9] There appears to be no association between disease activity and the development of obstetric complications, duration of labour, prematurity and fetal well-being.

Management

The management aims are to relieve pain and inflammation, to prevent joint destruction and to preserve or improve a patient's functional ability. Although drugs play an important role, non-drug therapy (e.g. rest, exercise, occupational therapy and psychological support) should always be considered.

Analgesia

- **Paracetamol is the analgesic of choice.**
- **Codeine may be used as an adjunct if required.**

Therapy for rheumatoid arthritis should begin with simple analgesia; paracetamol is the analgesic of choice. If pain is still present then codeine may be added. Although some epidemiological studies have suggested an association between opioids and specific congenital malformations,[10] most evidence suggests that therapeutic use in pregnancy has no adverse effect on fetal development. Opioids may be used at any stage of pregnancy for moderate to severe pain. Long-term *in utero* exposure may cause neonatal withdrawal symptoms (e.g. tremor, jitteriness and poor feeding),[11,12] and to prevent this opioids should be used sparingly in the last few weeks of pregnancy.

Lactation

Simple analgesics (paracetamol and codeine) are excreted into breast milk in small quantities,[13] and appear to be safe.

Non-steroidal anti-inflammatory agents (NSAIDs)

- Limited data do not suggest that exposure to NSAIDs in early pregnancy causes specific birth defects.
- If an NSAID is required, ibuprofen is preferred as it is the agent of choice in non-pregnant patients. Indomethacin should be avoided at any stage as it has been linked with problems more frequently than other agents.
- All NSAIDs should be avoided in the third trimester.

If simple analgesia does not relieve symptoms then NSAIDs may be considered. The use of NSAIDs in pregnancy has been investigated in depth with aspirin and indomethacin only.[6] There is no evidence of an increased risk of malformations with exposure to NSAIDs in early pregnancy.[8] Women who have inadvertently taken them may be reassured.

Adverse effects of NSAIDs

- The use of NSAIDs, even for short periods, after the 32nd week of pregnancy should be avoided due to a high incidence of premature closure of the ductus arteriosus.
- The use of NSAIDs, particularly during the third trimester of pregnancy, may cause a reduction in fetal urine output and oligohydramnios.
- NSAIDs may increase the incidence and duration of bleeding both in the fetus and mother during delivery. Pregnancy and labour may be prolonged due to prostaglandin inhibition.

The use of prostaglandin inhibitors such as NSAIDs or aspirin in late pregnancy may constrict the ductus arteriosus, leading to adverse fetal effects such as persistent pulmonary hypertension in the neonate and prolongation of pregnancy and labour.[8,14,15]

The fetal circulation is dependent on a patent or open ductus arteriosus, the blood vessel that allows blood to bypass the lungs. Prostaglandins (PGE_2 and prostacyclin) are the most important mediators of its vasodilation during fetal life. Maternal ingestion of aspirin and NSAIDs during the third trimester, even for short periods, has been associated with intrauterine closure of this blood vessel, leading to fetal and neonatal pulmonary hypertension and the syndrome of persistent fetal circulation.[6,16–21]

Prostaglandins also maintain the patency of the renal artery. Taken in pregnancy, prostaglandin inhibitors may lead to reduced fetal renal blood flow and a resultant fall in urine output. Oligohydramnios (a reduction in amniotic fluid) may result with subsequent fetal malformations.[22–26]

Studies of the efficacy of low-dose aspirin in the prevention of pre-eclampsia[27,28] and pregnancy-induced hypertension[29] have been reassuring with regard to its safety. However, analgesic doses may prolong spontaneous labour or increase the frequency of premature labour and should be avoided in late pregnancy.[30]

Prevention of NSAID-induced ulceration

> **All should be avoided in the first trimester. Cimetidine, omeprazole and misoprostol should be avoided. Ranitidine may be used.**

As many as 30% of long-term NSAID users develop gastric or duodenal ulcers.[31] The preferred drug for treatment or prophylaxis in pregnancy is ranitidine. Literature reports suggest that cimetidine has anti-androgenic effects in animals and although no problems in human pregnancy are known, its use cannot be recommended. Misoprostol should also be avoided in pregnancy. It can cause uterine contractions, and malformations have been reported following its unsuccessful use as an abortifacient.[32–36] There is insufficient information on omeprazole or other proton pump inhibitors to recommend their use in pregnancy.

Lactation

NSAIDs are excreted into breast milk in small quantities[13] and appear to be safe. Both cimetidine and ranitidine are excreted into breast milk but no neonatal effects have been reported with either agent. There is no information on the effects of misoprostol in lactation and it should be avoided.

Conclusion

There is no evidence that NSAIDs cause specific birth defects. However, all can interfere with pregnancy through their wide-ranging effects on prostaglandins. In women whose rheumatic disease justifies treatment, the lowest effective dose should be used. In general, high-potency agents, such as indomethacin, should be avoided at any stage and no NSAID should be used after 32 weeks gestation.

Disease-modifying anti-rheumatic drugs (DMARDs)

> **Sulphasalazine is the disease-modifying drug of choice in pregnancy.**

Active rheumatic disease not controlled with simple analgesia and NSAIDs may require the use of a disease-modifying anti-rheumatic drug (DMARD). Sulphasalazine is considered to be the agent of choice in pregnancy.[37] It is composed of sulphapyridine joined to 5-aminosalicylic acid (5-ASA). Sulphapyridine readily crosses the placenta while 5-ASA has limited placental transfer.[8] Experience in pregnancy is mainly derived from its use in inflammatory bowel disease,[38] where it has not been shown to increase the risk of malformations.[7] However, there are two potential problems with its use during the third trimester. Premature closure of the ductus arteriosus due to prostaglandin inhibition by 5-ASA is theoretically possible, although this problem has not been described after human exposure. There have been isolated reports of hyperbilirubinaemia and kernicterus in the neonate following exposure to sulphonamides.[39,40] This, once again, is a theoretical problem with sulphasalazine due to its sulphonamide component. Sulphasalazine may impair absorption of folate; however, there is no requirement to provide folic acid supplementation.

Antimalarials

> **Chloroquine and hydroxychloroquine should be avoided.**

Despite evidence that chloroquine for malaria prophylaxis in pregnancy is safe,[38] the safety of the higher doses required in rheumatic disease is unclear. Fetal toxicity has been described with high daily doses of chloroquine.[8] Malformations of the inner ear and other abnormalities were reported after chloroquine exposure in three siblings born of a mother with SLE.[41] Few data are available on the safety of hydroxychloroquine exposure during pregnancy.

In general, chloroquine and hydroxychloroquine should be avoided in pregnancy. However, since discontinuation of antimalarials in pregnant SLE patients may precipitate a flare with harmful consequences for mother and child, it seems reasonable to continue antimalarials in pregnant women with SLE.[42]

Lactation

Both chloroquine and hydroxychloroquine are found in small quantities in human milk.[38] Although there are few reports of adverse effects in breastfed infants, retinal damage is a theoretical risk.[1] Use of these drugs in breastfeeding women is therefore not recommended.

Gold salts

Gold salts, in high doses, have been shown to be teratogenic in animals.[38] There are no controlled studies of gold administration in human pregnancy. Available human data are conflicting and larger studies are needed to confirm whether or not there is a risk. Birth defects in humans have been attributed to gold,[6] and the compound was found in the liver and kidneys of an aborted human fetus.[43] A small number of studies suggest that gold is not teratogenic.[8] Due to the lack of safety data, the use of gold salts cannot be recommended in pregnancy. As these compounds have long half-lives, it has been suggested that pregnancy should be avoided for six months after treatment cessation.

Lactation

Up to 20% of an adult dose of gold may be found in breast milk and[44] gold has been shown to bind to the red blood cells of breastfed infants.[38] The theoretical possibility of toxicity precludes its use during breastfeeding.

Penicillamine

Patients with Wilson's disease and cystinuria treated with penicillamine have given birth to normal infants,[38] although exposure has been associated with the development of a generalised connective tissue defect in three infants.[8] In a study of 19 patients with rheumatoid arthritis, the only congenital anomaly reported was a ventricular septal defect (four patients had received penicillamine for the full term).[8] Penicillamine should be avoided in the treatment of rheumatic disease in pregnancy because safer alternatives exist.[38] Treatment should preferably be discontinued before a planned pregnancy or if a patient becomes pregnant while taking it. In Wilson's disease, however, the benefits of continued treatment may outweigh the small risk of teratogenicity.[42]

Lactation

Penicillamine is extensively protein bound and has a short half-life, so only small amounts should be present in breast milk. However, no studies in lactation have been carried out and the potential for toxicity precludes its use.

Immunosuppressants

Immunosuppressants are indicated in patients with severe, active, symptomatic and progressive joint disease that has failed to respond to other therapies. The timing of fetal exposure to immunosuppressants is critical. First-trimester use is most likely to produce congenital malformations or miscarriage. In the second and third trimesters, fetal growth and functional development can be impaired.[38] The long-term effects of immunosuppression on the children of mothers treated with these agents during pregnancy has not been established,[7] although interim results of one study are reassuring.[44] There is a possibility of chromosomal damage and a risk of carcinogenesis in later life. These drugs should always be stopped before conception (Tables 14.1 and 14.2), although the optimal timing of pregnancy after these drugs have been taken is not known.

Table 14.1: Anti-rheumatic and immunosuppressive drugs

Drug class	Withdrawal required before pregnancy?	Use during pregnancy
Non-steroidal anti-inflammatory drugs	No	Stop treatment at week 32 of gestation
Disease-modifying anti-rheumatic drugs	If possible	Most DMARDs should be avoided during pregnancy
Sulphasalazine	No	Drug of choice for second-line treatment
Gold compounds (sodium aurothiomalate, auranofin)	**Stop at least six months before conception**	Contraindicated
Antimalarials (e.g. chloroquine, hydroxychloroquine)	If possible	Avoid – except in SLE
Azathioprine	If possible	Avoid
Cyclosporin	If possible	Avoid
Penicillamine	If possible	Avoid – except in Wilson's disease
Cyclophosphamide	If possible	Contraindicated
Methotrexate	**Stop at least six months before conception**	Contraindicated
Leflunomide	Yes. Contraception must be used by men and women during and for two years after use	Contraindicated Teratogenic in animals

Table 14.2:   Recommendations for anti-rheumatic agents in lactation

Drug	Excreted in breast milk?	Safe to use in lactation?
Paracetamol	Small quantities	Yes
Codeine	Small quantities	Yes
NSAIDs: Ibuprofen Diclofenac Naproxen	Small quantities	Yes
Gold salts	Yes	No
Penicillamine	No information on excretion into breast milk	No
Corticosteroids	Small quantities	Yes – risk to infant is small[70]
Cytotoxic drugs	Yes	No
Cyclosporin	Yes	No
Antimalarials	Small quantities	No – not at treatment doses

Azathioprine

Azathioprine is an extensively used immunosuppressive. In pregnancy there is most experience of its use in renal or heart-transplant recipients and inflammatory bowel disease.[8,46,47] Neonatal bone marrow suppression has been noted.[6] Experience to date does not suggest that it increases the risk of malformations.[48,49] Due to the lack of conclusive safety data, it is not possible to recommend the routine use of azathioprine in pregnancy. Continued treatment may be considered appropriate, however, in some patients with SLE.

Methotrexate

Methotrexate, a folic acid antagonist, is increasingly used in severe rheumatoid and psoriatic arthritis. It is prescribed at lower doses than in chemotherapy regimens and is usually prescribed in combination with folic acid once a week. Methotrexate has been reported to cause abnormalities following first-trimester exposure as an abortifacient.[50,51] Limb and digital anomalies and neural tube defects have also been reported.[41] Most reports of methotrexate use during pregnancy are in women receiving chemotherapy, but available evidence suggests that there is a risk of fetal malformation even after exposure to low doses.[52,53] No increased incidence of congenital malformation has been found in offspring of women treated with methotrexate prior to conception.[54,55] As methotrexate is a folate antagonist, exposure before the neural tube closes (four weeks after conception) may be associated with an increased risk of neural tube defects.[56,57] Methotrexate should be discontinued before a planned pregnancy. There is some debate about the most appropriate interval between stopping treatment and attempting to conceive, but the *British National Formulary* currently advises a period of six months.

Cyclosporin

Cyclosporin is used in the treatment of various autoimmune and connective tissue diseases. It crosses the placenta and is found in the fetal circulation at concentrations of 10–50% of those reported in maternal blood.[5] Case reports of exposure in pregnancy do not suggest that it is a teratogen.[46,47,58–62] However, until more data are available it is difficult to be conclusive on its safety. Growth retardation has been reported after *in utero* cyclosporin exposure,[63] but the disease states being treated may have contributed to this problem. Cyclosporin is unlikely to be a teratogen and its use in pregnancy may be acceptable in some circumstances.[42]

Cyclophosphamide

Low-dose cyclophosphamide has been used to treat rheumatoid arthritis. Evidence suggests that there may be an increased risk of malformations.[52,53] Cyclophosphamide is contraindicated in pregnancy.

Lactation

Methotrexate, cyclophosphamide, azathioprine and cyclosporin are present in breast milk in low concentrations. They are all contraindicated in breastfeeding mothers due to the potential for immunosuppression, neutropenia and adverse effects on growth.

Corticosteroids

- **No evidence of increased risk of birth defects.**
- **Potential risk of neonatal adrenal suppression with long-term, high-dose steroid therapy. Following long-term, high-dose exposure to corticosteroids, neonates should be monitored for signs of adrenal suppression.**

Corticosteroids are used during pregnancy in asthma, idiopathic thrombocytopenia, inflammatory bowel disease and after transplantation.

They are also used to control joint inflammation and organ manifestations of rheumatic diseases. There is also considerable experience with short-term corticosteroid therapy for enhancing fetal lung maturity shortly before anticipated premature delivery.[64]

There is no evidence that exposure to corticosteroids leads to an increased risk of congenital malformations in humans.[49] Although some animal studies suggest an increased risk of oral clefts associated with corticosteroids, human studies have failed to demonstrate teratogenic or toxic effects.[64,65] Women taking long-term oral steroids should be monitored for pregnancy-induced glucose intolerance, hypertension and delayed fetal growth.[66] Long-term use of corticosteroids may cause intrauterine growth retardation and be associated with low birth weight.[8] This association may be a result of the effects of the disease on the course of the pregnancy. Rare cases of transient fetal adrenal suppression have been reported after high-dose corticosteroid exposure close to term.[64] There is no need for routine endocrine testing; however, it is important to monitor neonates closely for potential adrenal suppression after exposure *in utero* to high-dose corticosteroids.[38] On the evidence available there are no grounds for withholding corticosteroid therapy during pregnancy and the principles for prescribing them are the same as for non-pregnant women.

Lactation

In the doses used to treat rheumatic diseases there is little chance of an infant receiving appreciable amounts of prednisolone in breast milk. Breastfeeding is safe while taking corticosteroids (up to the equivalent of 40 mg prednisolone daily).

Summary

Pregnancy usually leads to an improvement in the symptoms of rheumatoid arthritis. Simple anti-inflammatory drugs and corticosteroids in low dosage probably do not produce any major problems. There is a lack of outcome data for most DMARDs in pregnancy. If possible, these agents should be stopped as soon as pregnancy is diagnosed, but the risk of disease flare through stopping a drug in well-controlled disease might be unacceptable. In women exposed inadvertently during early pregnancy, therapeutic abortion on the basis of drug exposure is probably unwarranted.

Immunosuppressant drugs should be avoided at all times except when the mother's health is at risk. The continued use of disease-remitting agents throughout pregnancy is probably not necessary and evidence of their safety is insufficient.

Osteoarthritis

Osteoarthritis (OA) features slow, progressive joint degeneration, which is usually monoarticular (less commonly polyarticular). The cause is unknown and the therapeutic goals are pain relief, increased mobility and reduction of disability. Therapeutic options are limited and mainly involve simple analgesics, NSAIDs and intra-articular corticosteroid injections for symptom relief. These approaches are also appropriate in pregnant women. Simple analgesics are the treatment of choice.

Carpal tunnel syndrome

Carpal tunnel syndrome is a common nerve compression problem and occurs in as many as 25% of pregnant women, normally between the fourth and ninth months of gestation. Treatment is symptomatic; a lightweight splint may be of benefit or perhaps local corticosteroid injections.[2]

Back pain

Back pain is one of the most common ailments in pregnancy, affecting almost 50% of women. It should be treated with rest, simple analgesics and, provided the previous recommendations are followed, NSAIDs (*see* p. 179).

Systemic lupus erythematosus (SLE)

> * **Active SLE during pregnancy is associated with both maternal and fetal problems.**
> * **SLE can affect an individual differently in successive pregnancies.**

SLE is a multisystem disease which most frequently presents in young women.[37] It affects between one in 2000 and one in 5000 pregnancies. The commonest findings in SLE are arthritis, rash, pleuropericarditis, fever, photosensitivity, lymphadenopathy, alopecia and Raynaud's phenomenon.[2] Typically an SLE patient has periods of disease exacerbation and remission, which occur at unpredictable intervals.

The major dilemma in treating pregnant women with SLE is that active disease is associated with both maternal and fetal problems.[2] Women with SLE in remission should, in most cases, remain on the same medication as treatment withdrawal may put the fetus at greater risk from active disease than from any adverse effects of medication.

Pregnancy and SLE

In women with quiescent disease at conception there is probably no change in the frequency of exacerbations; disease flare tends to occur in the first trimester or post-partum.[9] Systemic lupus erythematosus does not necessarily affect an individual in the same way during successive pregnancies.[67] Women with active disease at conception have an increased risk of fetal loss. Disease exacerbations may cause haemolytic anaemia, thrombocytopenic purpura, polyserositis or renal damage. These may complicate pregnancy; renal disease predisposes patients to hypertension/pre-eclampsia; anaemia may affect fetal well-being (including growth retardation) and thrombocytopenia may, rarely, be transmitted to the fetus.[2] Exacerbations involving single-organ systems are more common.

Fetal death, intrauterine growth retardation and prematurity are common in women with SLE[2] and their frequency is related to disease severity. A condition known as neonatal lupus syndrome (NLS) may occur in infants born to some mothers with SLE.[68–70] The syndrome consists of a combination of haematological problems (thrombocytopenia and haemolytic anaemia), photosensitive rash and congenital complete heart block.

Management

There is no requirement for routine prophylaxis of exacerbations of SLE in pregnancy; treat symptomatically. Paracetamol and NSAIDs are frequently used for joint and neurological involvement. Rashes may be treated with topical or systemic corticosteroids.[37] Corticosteroids are the treatment of choice for managing disease exacerbations (e.g. thrombocytopenia and anaemia).[66] Low-dose aspirin may be used to prevent pre-eclampsia in patients with renal disease.* All women with SLE who wish to become pregnant require close monitoring by both an obstetrician and a rheumatologist.

---

*Although initial studies and meta-analysis suggested benefit, recent large randomised controlled trials have failed to show benefit, even in women at high risk of pre-eclampsia.[71,72] There is some suggestion, however, that it may be useful in women with a history of early onset pre-eclampsia in a previous pregnancy and some specialists may recommend it in this situation.

References

1 Needs CJ and Brooks PM (1985) Anti-rheumatic medication in pregnancy. *Br J Rheumatol.* **24**: 282–90.

2 Lockshin MD and Druzin ML (1995) Rheumatic disease. In *Medical Disorders During Pregnancy* (2nd edn) (eds WM Barron and MD Lindheimer). Mosby Year Books, St Louis.

3 Nelson JL, Koepsell TD, Dugowson CE *et al.* (1993) Fecundity before disease onset in women with rheumatoid arthritis. *Arthrit Rheumat.* **36**(1): 7–14.

4 Del Junco DJ, Annegers JF, Coulam CB *et al.* (1989) The relationship between rheumatoid arthritis and reproductive function. *Br J Rheumatol.* **28**(I): 33.

5 Ostensen M and Husby G (1983) A prospective clinical study of the effect of pregnancy on rheumatoid arthritis and ankylosing spondylitis. *Arthrit Rheumat.* **26**(9): 1155–9.

6 Witter FR (1993) Clinical pharmacokinetics in the treatment of rheumatoid arthritis in pregnancy. *Clin Pharmacokinet.* **25**(6): 444–9.

7 Kean WF and Buchanan WW (1990) Pregnancy and rheumatoid disease. *Bailliere's Clin Rheumatol.* **4**(1): 125–40.

8 Ostensen M (1994) Optimisation of anti-rheumatic drug treatment in pregnancy. *Clin Pharmacokinet.* **27**(6): 486–503.

9 Nicholas NS (1988) Rheumatic dieases in pregnancy. *Br J Hosp Med.* **39**(1): 50–3.

10 Heinonen OP, Slone D and Shapiro S (eds) (1977) *Birth Defects and Drugs in Pregnancy.* PSG Publishing Company, Inc.

11 Mangurten HH and Benawra R (1980) Neonatal codeine withdrawal in infants of non-addicted mothers. *Pediatrics.* **65**(1): 159–60.

12 Chasnoff IJ *et al* (1984) Perinatal addiction: the effects of maternal narcotic and non-narcotic substance abuse on the fetus and neonate. *Natl Inst Drug Abuse Res Monogr Ser.* 49: 220–6.

13 Anderson PO (1991) Therapy review: breastfeeding. *Clin Pharm.* **10**: 602–15.

14 Rudolph AM (1981) The effects of non-steroidal anti-inflammatory compounds on fetal circulation and pulmonary function. *Obstet Gynecol.* **58**: S63–S67.

15 Prasad RNV (1982) Prostaglandin synthetase inhibitors and their effects on the fetus and the newborn. *Ann Acad Med.* **11**(4): 513–20.

16 van den Veyver, Moise KJ Jr, Ou CN *et al.* (1993) The effect of gestational age and fetal indomethacin levels on the incidence of constriction of the fetal ductus arteriosus. *Obstet Gynecol.* **82**: 500–3.

17 Eronen M (1993) The hemodynamic effects of antenatal indomethacin and a beta-sympathomimetic agent on the fetus and the newborn: a randomised study. *Pediatr Res.* **33**(6): 615–19.

18 Moise KJ Jr, Huhta JC, Sharif DS *et al.* (1988) Indomethacin in the treatment of premature labor: effects on the fetal ductus arteriosus. *N Engl J Med.* **319**: 327–31.

19 Norton ME (1993) Neonatal complications after the administration of indomethacin for pre-term labor. *N Engl J Med.* **329**: 1602–7.

20 Moise KJ (1993) Effect of advancing gestational age on the frequency of fetal ductal constriction in association with maternal indomethacin use. *Am J Obstet Gynecol.* **168**: 1350–3.

21 Wilkinson AR, Aynsley-Green A, Mitchell MD *et al.* (1979) Persistent pulmonary hypertension and abnormal prostaglandin E levels in pre-term infants after maternal treatment with naproxen. *Arch Dis Child.* **54**: 942–5.

22 Voyer LE, Drut R and Mendez JH (1994) Fetal renal maldevelopment with oligohydramnios following maternal use of piroxicam. *Pediatr Nephrol.* **8**(5): 592–4.

23 Gloor JM (1993) Prenatal maternal indomethacin use resulting in prolonged neonatal insufficiency. *J Perinatol.* **XIII**(6): 4257.

24 van der Heijden BJ, Carlus C, Narcy F *et al.* (1994) Persistent anuria, neonatal death and renal microcystic lesions after prenatal exposure to indomethacin. *Am J Obstet Gynecol.* **171**: 617–23.

25 Uslu T, Ozcan FS and Aydin C (1992) Oligohydramnios induced by maternal indomethacin therapy. *Int J Clin Pharm Ther Toxicol.* **30**(7): 230–2.

26 Kirshon B, Moise KJ Jr, Mari G *et al.* (1991) Long-term indomethacin therapy decreases fetal urine output and results in oligohydramnios. *Am J Perinatol.* **8**(2): 86–8.

27 CLASP (Collaborative Low-dose Aspirin Study in Pregnancy) Collaborative Group. (1994) CLASP: a randomised trial of low-dose aspirin for the prevention and treatment of pre-eclampsia among 9364 pregnant women. *Lancet.* **343**: 619–29.

28 Sibai BM, Caritis SN, Thom E *et al.* (1993) Prevention of pre-eclampsia with low-dose aspirin in healthy, nulliparous pregnant women. *N Engl J Med.* **329**: 1213–18.

29 Imperiale TF and Petrulis AS (1991) A meta-analysis of low-dose aspirin for the prevention of pregnancy-induced hypertensive disease. *JAMA.* **266**(2): 261–5.

30 Lewis RB and Schulman JD (1973) Influence of acetylsalicylic acid, an inhibitor of prostaglandin synthesis, on the duration of human gestation and labour. *Lancet.* **2**: 1159–61.

31 Miller DR (1992) Treatment of non-steroidal anti-inflammatory drug-induced gastropathy. *Clin Pharm.* **11**: 690–704.

32 Coelho HLL, Teixeira AC, Santos AP *et al.* (1993) Misoprostol and illegal abortion in Fortaleza, Brazil. *Lancet.* **341**: 1261–3.

33 Castilla EE and Orioli IM (1994) Teratogenicity of misoprostol: data from the Latin-American Collaborative Study of Congenital Malformations (ECLAMC). *Am J Med Genet.* **51**: 161–2.

34 Shepard TH (1995) Mobius syndrome after misoprostol: a possible teratogenic mechanism. *Lancet.* **346**: 780.

35 Fonseca W, Alencar AJ, Pereira RM *et al.* (1993) Congenital malformation of the scalp and cranium after failed first-trimester abortion attempt with misoprostol. *Clin Dysmorphol.* **2**: 76–80.

36 Gonzalez CH, Vargas FR, Perez AB *et al.* (1993) Limb deficiency with or without Mobius sequence, in seven Brazilian children, associated with misoprostol use in the first trimester of pregnancy. *Am J Med Genet.* **47**: 59–64.

37 de Swiet M (1995) Systemic lupus erythematosus and other connective tissue diseases. In *Medical Disorders in Obstetric Practice* (3rd edn) (ed M de Swiet). Blackwell Science, Oxford.

38 Preston S and Needs C (1990) Guidelines on the use of anti-rheumatic drugs in women during pregnancy and child-bearing age. *Bailliere's Clin Rheumatol.* **4**(3): 687–98.

39 Lucey JF and Driscoll TJ (1959) Hazard to newborn infants of administration of long-acting sulfonamides to pregnant women. *Pediatrics.* **24**: 498–9.

40 Dunn PM *et al.* (1964) The possible relationship between the maternal administration of sulphamethoxypyridine and hyperbilirubinaemia in the newborn. *J Obstet Gynecol Br Commonwealth.* **71**: 128–31.

41 Briggs GG, Freeman RK and Yaffe SJ (1994) *Drugs in Pregnancy and Lactation* (4th edn). Williams & Wilkins, Baltimore.

42 Ostensen M and Ramsey Goldman R (1998) Treatment of inflammatory rheumatic disorders in pregnancy. What are the safest treatment options? *Drug Safety.* **19**(5): 389–410.

43 Rocker I and Henderson WJ (1976) Transfer of gold from mother to fetus. *Lancet.* **2**: 1246.

44 Lawrence RA (1994) *Breastfeeding: a guide for the medical profession* (4th edn). Mosby, St Louis.

45 Ramsay-Goldman R, Mientus JM, Kutzer JE *et al.* (1993) Pregnancy outcome in women with systemic lupus erythematosus treated with immunosuppressive drugs. *J Rheumatol.* **20**: 1152–7.

46 Armenti VT, Ahlswede KM, Ahlswede BA *et al.* (1994) National transplantation pregnancy registry: outcomes of 154 pregnancies in cyclosporine-treated female kidney transplant recipients. *Transplantation.* **57**: 502–6.

47 Scott JR, Wagoner LE, Olsen SL *et al.* (1993) Pregnancy in heart-transplant recipients: management and outcome. *Obstet Gynecol.* **82**: 324–7.

48 Alstead EM, Ritchie JK, Lennard-Jones JE *et al.* (1990) Safety of azathioprine in pregnancy in inflammatory bowel disease. *Gastroenterology.* **99**: 443–6.

49 Roubenoff R, Hoyt J, Petri M *et al.* (1988) Effects of anti-inflammatory and immunosuppressive drugs on pregnancy and fertility. *Sem Arthrit Rheumat.* **18**(2): 88–110.

50 Milunsky A, Graef JW, Gaynor MF *et al.* (1968) Methotrexate-induced congenital malformations. *J Pediatr.* 790–5.

51 Warkany J (1978) Aminopterin and methotrexate: folic acid deficiency. *Teratology.* **17**: 353–8.

52 Stuijit CCM *et al.* (1994) Chemotherapy during pregnancy: a report based on recent literature data. *J Drug Devel.* **6**(3): 99–106.

53 Blatt J, Mulvihill JJ, Ziegler JL *et al.* (1980) Pregnancy outcome following cancer chemotherapy. *Am J Med.* **69**: 828–32.

54 Rustin GJS, Booth M, Dent J *et al.* (1984) Pregnancy after cytotoxic chemotherapy for gestational trophoblastic tumours. *BMJ.* **288**: 103–6.

55 Kozlowski RD, Steinbrunner JV, MacKenzie AH *et al.* (1990) Outcome of first-trimester exposure to low-dose methotrexate in eight patients with rheumatic disease. *Am J Med.* **88**: 589–92.

56 Moore KL and Persaud TVN (1993). The nervous system. In *The Developing Human: clinically orientated embryology* (5th edn) (eds KL Moore and TVN Persand), pp. 385–422. WB Saunders and Co, Philadelphia.

57 Donnenfeld AE, Pastuszak A, Noah JS *et al.* (1994) Methotrexate exposure prior to, and during, pregnancy. *Teratology.* **49**: 79–81.

58 Baruch Y, Weiner Z, Enat R *et al.* (1993) Pregnancy after liver transplantation. *Int J Gynecol Obstet.* **41**: 273–6.

59 Scantlebury V, Gordon R, Tzakis A *et al.* (1990) Childbearing after liver transplantation. *Transplantation.* **49**: 317–21.

60 Haugen G, Fauchald P, Sodal G *et al.* (1991) Pregnancy outcome in renal allograft recipients: influence of ciclosporin A. *Eur J Obstet Gynecol Reprod Biol.* **39**: 25–9.

61 Ville Y, Fernandez H, Samuel D *et al.* (1993) Pregancy in liver transplant recipients: course and outcome in 19 cases. *Am J Obstet Gynecol.* **168**: 896–902.

62 Al-Khader AA, Absy M, al-Hasani MK *et al.* (1988) Successful pregnancy in renal transplant recipients treated with cyclosporine. *Transplantation.* **45**(5): 987–8.

63 Huynh LA and Min DI (1994) Outcomes of pregnancy and the management of immunosuppressive agents to minimize fetal risks in organ transplant patients. *Ann Pharmacother.* **28**: 1355–7.

64 Rayburn WF (1992) Glucocorticoid therapy for rheumatic diseases: maternal, fetal and breastfeeding considerations. *Am J Reprod Immunol.* **28**: 138–40.

65 Fraser FC and Sajoo A (1995) Teratogenic potential of corticosteroids in humans. *Teratology.* **51**: 45–6.

66 Buyon JP (1990) Systemic lupus erythematosus and the maternal-fetal dyad. *Bailliere's Clin Rheumatol.* **4**(1): 85–103.

67 Estes D and Larson DL (1965) Systemic lupus eeythematosus and pregnancy. *Clin Obstet Gynecol.* **8**: 307–21.

68 Buyon JP, Winchester RJ, Slade SG *et al.* (1993) Identification of mothers at risk for congenital heart block and other neonatal lupus syndromes in their children. *Arthrit Rheumat.* **36**(9): 1263–73.

69 Lockshin MD, Bonfa E, Elkon K *et al.* (1988) Neonatal lupus risk to newborns of mothers with systemic lupus erythematosus. *Arthrit Rheumat.* **31**(6): 697–701.

70 Bennett PN (1988) *Drugs and Human Lactation.* Elsevier, Oxford.

71 Sibai BM (1996) Treatment of hypertension in pregnant women. *N Engl J Med.* **335**: 257–65.

72 Caritis S *et al.* (1998) Low-dose aspirin to prevent pre-eclampsia in women at high risk. *N Engl J Med.* **338**: 701–5.

CHAPTER FIFTEEN

Skin disorders

Elizabeth Bardolph and Richard Ashton

Introduction

Pregnancy can affect the largest organ in the body – the skin – in a number of differing and sometimes unpredictable ways. Many of the changes are common and unremarkable, for instance pigmentation of the nipples, areola and external genitalia. There are some conditions which alter with pregnancy and others which occur as a result of the gravid state. The principles of therapeutic treatment are primarily dependent on safety for the expectant mother and the fetus. The cosmetic effect of skin disease on the mother's self-esteem must also be considered.

In general, the use of systemic drugs is best avoided, although there are some situations where their use is appropriate and these will be discussed later. Most topical agents are not absorbed to the extent that blood levels sufficient to affect the growth or development of the fetus are achieved. However, this does not mean that all topical treatments may be safely used in pregnant women. Fetal abnormalities have been attributed to topical exposures[1,2] and due caution is needed, particularly with retinoids, but also with topical administration of any agent that is known to have teratogenic potential after systemic use.

This chapter will discuss the treatment of common diseases such as eczema and psoriasis in pregnancy and then the group of skin diseases occurring specifically during pregnancy.

Common skin disorders unrelated to pregnancy

Eczema

Eczema and dermatitis are terms that are interchangeable and refer to inflammation of the skin with specific histological features such as oedema of the epidermis (spongiosis), thickening of the epidermis and an inflammatory cell infiltrate within the dermis. Clinically, eczema is recognised as poorly defined erythematous papules, patches and plaques with exudate, crusting or scale. The commonest form is atopic eczema, presenting usually in childhood but in around 5% persisting into adult life. This is characterised by flexural eczema which in severe cases becomes generalised, with severe itching and scratching and lichenification.

Atopic eczema may worsen during pregnancy in some patients, and improve in others.

Effects on breastfeeding

- Breastfeeding may be a problem when eczema affects the nipples (as it often does). The nipples become cracked and painful, and there may be secondary infection with staphylococci. Treatment will be required to enable breastfeeding to take place. Application of steroid creams or ointments is unlikely to pose problems to the feeding baby.
- Eczema herpeticum is due to infection of eczematous skin by the herpes simplex virus. Rarely it may become systemic and affect mother and fetus.[3]

Treatment of atopic eczema

- Regular application of an emollient (e.g. aqueous cream, oily cream, Diprobase, E45 cream etc.).
- Aqueous cream or emulsifying ointment as soap substitutes.
- Mild to moderate topical corticosteroids will be required for treatment of eczematous skin. Ointment is generally better than cream on dry skin. The usual problem is undertreatment due to fear of use of topical steroids. It is best to use steroids intensively for short periods of time, five to seven days, with intervening periods of emollient use (two to three days).

There has been concern about the potential for corticosteroids to cause fetal harm. This arose mainly from observations that administration to pregnant animals caused abnormalities, including cleft lip and palate and effects on brain growth and development.[4] However, in humans there is no convincing evidence that systemic corticosteroids cause an increase in congenital abnormalities.[4,5] Topical corticosteroids may be used during pregnancy, but high-potency agents (such as clobelasol propionate 0.05%) should be avoided if possible.

- Potassium permanganate (1:1000 solution) diluted to a light pink colour in a bath or as wet dressings if the eczema is acute or weepy. This dries up the exudate and unless this is done application of other topical agents is ineffective.

- Systemic antihistamines. A sedative antihistamine is preferred, for example chlorpheniramine or promethazine.[6–9] Non-sedating antihistamines (*see* urticaria, p. 200) should only be used if the above produce unacceptable drowsiness.[10–12]

    Published literature on pregnancy outcome after exposure to antihistamines does not suggest that any of these agents are associated with a high risk of teratogenic effects.[6] Chlorpheniramine is the antihistamine of choice; published data on pregnancy outcome in several thousand women show no evidence of an increased fetal risk.[7,8] Data for promethazine and diphenhydramine indicate that these drugs are unlikely to pose a substantial risk.[8,9]

- If eczema herpeticum occurs during pregnancy, systemic aciclovir may be given. This is a particularly distressing condition resulting in pain and discomfort and generally merits hospital admission. The available data do not suggest that aciclovir exposure is associated with increased fetal risk[13] and the potential risks of treatment are outweighed by the benefit of avoiding an intrauterine herpes simplex infection.[3]

- Gamolenic acid should be used with caution as there is very little information on its effects on the fetus. However, there is no evidence that it is harmful.

Psoriasis

Psoriasis is a chronic skin disease, commonly presenting between the ages of 15 and 25 and affecting around 1–2% of the population. Most cases are mild with well-circumscribed scaly erythematous plaques on the elbows, knees and less often on lower legs, scalp and elsewhere. Scratching the scaly plaques results in the production of detachable, fine, silver scaling, a useful diagnostic test.

Effects on pregnancy

The majority of pregnant patients experience a change in their psoriasis during pregnancy and post-partum. The condition usually improves due to changes in circulating oestrogens and progesterone which alter the immune system.[14]

Treatment

Topical agents safe to use in pregnancy

*   Emollients.
*   Salicylic acid ointment 2–5% to remove scale and hydrate skin. Although systemic absorption of salicylates is likely, there is no evidence that this would result in fetal harm. Experience with the use of low-dose aspirin in the prevention and treatment of pre-eclampsia suggests that it is reasonably safe[15] and by extrapolation topical salicylates are unlikely to cause problems. Nevertheless, prolonged or extensive use should be avoided if possible, particularly near term.

Use with caution

*   Dithranol cream may be used, but it can cause local irritation as well as staining. There are inadequate data on the effects of dithranol in human pregnancy. It may have antimitotic activity which is a theoretical concern.
*   Dithranol in Lassar's paste for large, thick plaques.
*   Refined tar (coal tar solution) is contained in many proprietary products. There is currently some concern about the potential carcinogenicity of coal tar.[16]
*   Ultraviolet light (UVB).
*   Calcipotriol is a vitamin D analogue; about 5% is absorbed after topical application. It should not be used on the face, and the hands should be washed carefully after application as it may cause irritation. Its safety in pregnancy has not been established. Hypercalcaemia and signs of hypervitaminosis D may occur as a result of systemic absorption if treatment exceeds the recommended dose (100 g per week). Safety in breastfeeding has not been established.
*   Tacalcitol is similar to calcipotriol. Its safety in pregnancy has not been established.

Contraindicated drugs

- Retinoids are teratogenic.[17] Acitretin (Neotigason) is a systemic retinoid used extensively in the treatment of psoriasis. It reduces scaling and after two months produces considerable improvement in many patients. All women of child-bearing potential who are treated with acitretin must use an effective contraceptive for at least one month before, and during, treatment and for at least two years after a course of the drug. *In utero* retinoid exposure is believed to affect the cephalic neural crest, resulting in an increased rate of spontaneous abortion and congenital malformations that are mainly cranial/facial, cardiac and thymic.[18] Most dermatologists would not prescribe acitretin for psoriasis in women until they are unlikely to have any more children.
- Tazarotene is a new topical retinoid for use in moderate plaque psoriasis. Systemic absorption of the active metabolite is minimal.[19] As with other retinoids, tazarotene is contraindicated in pregnancy. It is also contraindicated in breastfeeding.
- Methotrexate must not be given to women who are pregnant or planning a pregnancy. It is a folate antagonist which impairs dihydrofolate reductase and interferes with purine production. Methotrexate is believed to be retained in human tissues for long periods. Experience with its use to terminate pregnancy and in the treatment of cancer suggests that it has teratogenic effects.[20,21] There is a risk of fetal malformation even with low-dose therapy.[22] Pregnancy should be avoided if either partner is receiving the drug. Men and women should wait a minimum of six months after stopping treatment before attempting to conceive.[23]
- Methotrexate is excreted in breast milk and its use in breastfeeding mothers is contraindicated.
- PUVA involves the combination of a psoralen tablet with UVA exposure two hours later. There are theoretical reasons for not taking psoralens while pregnant or breastfeeding.[24]
- Cyclosporin – available data on pregnancy outcome after exposure, mainly in women who have had organ transplants, suggest that fetal risk is low.[8] However, it should be avoided in pregnant women with psoriasis, as experience is limited.

Acne

Effects on pregnancy

The increased levels of oestrogens in pregnancy reduce the influence of testosterone on the sebaceous follicle and are likely to improve acne. However, acne may behave unpredictably[25] and can sometimes become worse.

Treatment

Topical agents safe to use in pregnancy

- Topical agents which remove keratin and unblock the duct, such as benzoyl peroxide (5%, 10%), may be used.[26]
- Topical antibiotics are not absorbed into the bloodstream. Topical erythromycin and clindamycin are not known to be harmful so may be used. Topical tetracycline is best avoided.

Contraindicated drugs

- Systemic tetracyclines, e.g tetracycline, oxytetracycline, minocycline and doxycycline, are contraindicated in pregnancy due to deposition in growing bones and teeth and resultant risk of fetal abnormalities.[7] The deciduous teeth begin to calcify at around five or six months *in utero* so exposure after this time may lead to staining. There is inadequate evidence that exposure to tetracyclines in early pregnancy is associated with an increased risk of fetal abnormality.[7,26,27] Inadvertent exposure during the first few weeks of pregnancy should not be regarded as an indication for termination of pregnancy; a detailed ultrasound scan may be offered.
- Tetracyclines should be avoided in breastfeeding, although the potential for adverse effects is minimised by chelation of the drug with calcium in milk. Short-term use may be reasonable in some situations.
- All retinoids, including isotretinoin, topical tretinoin (retinoic acid) and adapelene, must not be given to women of child-bearing potential. A pregnancy test must be carried out in all women of child-bearing potential before oral isotretinoin is prescribed. Effective contraception must be practised for at least one month before, during and for at least one month after treatment.[28] A recent survey of dermatologists in Scotland found that pregnancy tests were not always carried out before initiating therapy and that the possibility of sexual activity in girls under 16 years was not always recognised.[29] Isotretinoin is the most potent teratogen in routine use today and it is vital that the prescribing recommendations are adhered to in order to avoid inadvertent exposure during pregnancy. Women should be counselled about the risks and ideally given written information

about the need to avoid pregnancy during, and for one month after, treatment. If a woman does become pregnant while taking oral isotretinoin she should be referred to an obstetrician for specialist counselling and advice.

Whether topical retinoids are associated with teratogenic effects is less clear.[30] There have been case reports of birth defects after topical exposure[1,2] but more recent epidemiological studies are reassuring.[31,32] A retrospective case-control study comparing pregnancy outcome in 215 women exposed to topical tretinoin with a control group found no association with abnormalities typical of retinoid exposure.[31] A prospective study comparing a cohort of 94 exposed women with a control group found no difference in the rates of live births, miscarriages or elective terminations of pregnancy.[32] There was also no difference in the incidence of major malformations in live births. Women who are inadvertently exposed to topical retinoids during pregnancy should probably have a detailed scan.

- The anti-androgen cyproterone acetate may cause feminisation of the male fetus but is generally only given with oestrogen as an oral contraceptive.

Urticaria

Urticaria or hives is the result of dermal oedema seen clinically as erythematous wheals. The individual lesions should last less than 24 hours, although new lesions appear continuously. Although commonly assumed to be an 'allergy', unless the precipitating factor is obvious and immediate, the cause is likely to be unknown. Ingestion of aspirin, codeine or tartrazine may precipitate an acute attack.

Effects on pregnancy
None.

Treatment
Systemic antihistamines may be used either to control an acute episode or prophylactically to reduce recurrent lesions.

Published literature on pregnancy outcome after exposure to antihistamines does not suggest that any of these agents are associated with a high risk of teratogenic effects.[6] Chlorpheniramine is the antihistamine of choice; published data on pregnancy outcome in several thousand women shows no evidence of an increased fetal risk.[7,8] Data for promethazine and diphenhydramine indicate that these drugs are unlikely to pose a substantial risk.[8,9]

There is much less experience with newer, non-sedating antihistamines, such as terfenadine, cetirizine and loratadine, and consequently these should be avoided. However, the limited available data do not suggest an association with birth defects so women exposed inadvertently may be reassured.[6,10,11] Astemizole (now discontinued) has caused defects in animal studies and is contraindicated in pregnant women.[12]

Summary

Tables 15.1 and 15.2 summarise the safety in pregnancy and lactation of drugs prescribed for common skin disorders.

Table 15.1:   Safety in pregnancy of drugs prescribed for common skin disorders

Disorder	Permitted drugs	Use with caution	Contraindicated
Eczema	Emollient Aqueous cream Topical corticosteroids	Aciclovir Gamolenic acid	
Psoriasis	Emollient Salicylic acid	Dithranol Tar Calcipotriol Tacalcitol	All systemic drugs, including retinoids, methotrexate, PUVA, cyclosporin
Urticaria	Chlorpheniramine Promethazine	Terfenadine Cetirizine Loratadine	Astemizole
Acne	Benzoyl peroxide Topical erythromycin	Topical tetracycline	Systemic tetracyclines All retinoids

Table 15.2:   Safety in breastfeeding of drugs prescribed for common skin disorders

Drug	Safety in breastfeeding	Comments
May be used		
Emollients	Safe	
Antihistamines – non-sedating (e.g. terfenadine, cetirizine, loratidine)	No evidence of harmful effects. Contraindicated in prescribing information. Cetirizine or loratadine preferred if non-sedating drug required.	Terfenadine not recommended due to potential for cardiac arrhythmias if elevated plasma levels occur.
Antihistamines – sedating (e.g. chlorpheniramine, promethazine, trimeprazine)	Excreted in breast milk. Generally considered safe.	Sedative effects in the infant are possible. Avoid clemastine.
Systemic corticosteroids	Excreted in breast milk. Doses of up to 40 mg daily unlikely to cause systemic effects.	High doses may lead to adrenal suppression in the infant.
Topical corticosteroids	Harmful effects unlikely with use at recommended doses.	Safe.
Coal tar	No evidence of harmful effects.	
Dithranol	No evidence of harmful effects.	
Benzoyl peroxide	No evidence of harmful effects.	
Antibiotics, topical	No evidence of harmful effects.	
Gamolenic acid	No evidence of harmful effects.	
Use with caution		
Tetracyclines	Avoid due to potential for adverse effects on developing teeth and bones.	Absorption in the infant likely to be low due to chelation with calcium in milk.
Vitamin D analogues (calcipotriol, tacalcitol)	Avoid excessive use due to potential for hypercalcaemia.	Inadequate evidence of safety.
Do not use		
Retinoids (oral or topical)	Contraindicated.	
Cyclosporin	Contraindicated.	Experience limited.
Methotrexate	Contraindicated.	

Skin disorders as a result of pregnancy

Pruritus gravidarum

Itching in pregnancy may be a distressing physiological symptom and the aetiology is probably multifactorial. Oestrogen impairs the transport of bile to the bile canaliculi, leading to an increase in circulating bile salts. Prostaglandins may reduce the threshold for pruritis. Liver function should always be checked to exclude cholestasis.

Treatment

Antihistamines (chlorpheniramine) and soothing emollients, such as 0.5% menthol in aqueous cream, may be helpful.

Polymorphic eruption of pregnancy

This is also known as pruritic urticarial papules and plaques of pregnancy (PUPPP), toxic erythema of pregnancy or toxic rash of pregnancy. This is the most common rash in pregnancy, with an incidence of about one in 200 pregnancies.[33] It typically affects primigravidas and the rash most commonly develops during the third trimester or post-partum.

Cause

It is possibly related to abdominal distension during pregnancy. This has been hypothesised because of the association with increased maternal weight gain and increased newborn weight, and disease in twin pregnancies tends to be more severe.[34]

Diagnosis
- Small erythematous urticarial papules which coalesce to form large plaques.
- Starts on the abdominal striae but can spread to the arms and legs.
- The rash is extremely itchy.

Effects on pregnancy
- It is very distressing for the mother because of the intense itching, which can result in loss of sleep.

- It fades two to three weeks post-partum and subsequent pregnancies are unaffected.
- The baby is not affected.

Drug treatment

- Topical calamine lotion or topical steroid twice daily may help.
- A brief tapering course of systemic corticosteroids will provide relief.
- Oral chlorpheniramine 4 mg four times a day may be used, but evidence of efficacy is limited.
- It is important to assure the patient that the condition is not serious, will not harm the baby and disappears at, or soon after, birth.

Pemphigoid (herpes) gestationitis

This rare condition (occurring in one in 60 000 pregnancies) usually develops in the second or third trimester or in the immediate post-partum.[33] It bears no relation to the viral condition other than blistering is present. It is very itchy and the lesions, although urticated papules and plaques initially, become bullous and may look identical to bullous pemphigoid. The eruption often starts around the umbilicus and spreads to the thighs and then the limbs.

Causes

It is an acquired autoimmune bullous dermatosis disease with autoantibodies (IgG) in the basement layer of the skin. Hormonal factors are involved in the aetiology.

Diagnosis

It is distinguished from polymorphic rash of pregnancy by the presence of large bullae and immunofluorescence on skin biopsy.

Effects on pregnancy

- The extreme itchiness may prevent sleep at night and cause distress during the day.
- In extreme cases the patient may be ill with fever, rigors and vomiting.
- Occasionally the baby may be born with the same rash.
- There is a risk of low birth weight in the baby.

- May take weeks to clear post-partum.
- It tends to recur in subsequent pregnancies and may become more severe.

Drug treatment

- Ice packs on the itchy areas will help in the short term.
- Mild cases may respond to moderately potent topical steroids. If the patient is near term, potent topical steroids (such as clobetasol propionate) may help. Otherwise systemic steroids, such as prednisolone 20–80 mg daily, will be necessary for the bullous lesions. The dose may be reduced once the blistering is under control.[34]
- Systemic antibiotics may be needed if superinfection of bullous lesions occurs.

Prurigo of pregnancy

This condition (also known as prurigo gravidarum or early-onset prurigo of pregnancy) affects about one in 300 pregnancies.[33] Its presenting feature is very itchy skin with excoriations caused by scratching. The condition usually occurs at the end of the second or beginning of the third trimester.

Causes

It is thought to be due to pruritus gravidarum occurring in a patient with atopy.

Effects on pregnancy

- Fetus prognosis is normal.
- The condition ceases post-partum but can recur during subsequent pregnancies.

Drug treatment

- Symptomatic treatment tends to be unsatisfactory.
- Emollients, such as E45 or oily cream, or systemic antihistamines, such as chlorpheniramine or promethazine, may help.

Contraindicated drugs

Systemic steroids.

Summary

Table 15.3: Treatment of skin disorders occurring as a result of pregnancy

Disorder	Drugs of choice	Use with caution	Contraindicated
Pruritus gravidarum	0.5% menthol in aqueous cream Chlorpheniramine		
Polymorphic eruption (PUPPP)	Topical steroids Chlorpheniramine	Systemic steroids	
Prurigo gravidarum	Emollient Chlorpheniramine		Systemic steroids
Pemphigoid gestationis	Topical steroids	Systemic steroids	

References

1   Camera G and Pregliasco P (1992) Ear malformation in baby born to mother using tretinoin cream. *Lancet.* **339**: 687.

2   Lipson AH, Collins F and Webster WS (1993) Multiple congenital defects associated with maternal use of topical tretinoin. *Lancet.* **341**: 1352–3.

3   Wollenberg A and Degitz K (1995) Eczema herpeticatum in graviditae. *Deutshe Medizinische Wochenschrift.* **120**(41): 1395–8.

4   Fraser FC and Sajoo A (1995) Teratogenic potential of corticosteroids in humans. *Teratology.* **51**: 45–6.

5   CSM/MCA (1998) Systemic corticosteroids in pregnancy and lactation. *Current Problems in Pharmacovigilance.* **24**: 9.

6   Schatz M, Zeiger RS, Harden K *et al.* (1997) The safety of asthma and allergy medications during pregnancy. *J Aller Clin Immunol.* **100**: 301–6.

7   Briggs GG, Freeman RK and Yaffe SJ (1994) *Drugs in Pregnancy and Lactation: a reference guide to fetal and neonatal risk* (4th edn). Williams and Wilkins, Baltimore.

8   Friedman JM and Polifka JE (1996) *The Effects of Drugs on the Fetus and Nursing Infant: a handbook for health care professionals.* Johns Hopkins University Press, Baltimore.

9   Aselton P, Jick H, Milunsky A *et al.* (1985) First-trimester drug use and congenital disorders. **65**: 451–5.

10 Schick B, Hom M, Librizzi R *et al.* (1994) Terfenadine exposure in early pregnancy. *Teratology.* **49**(5): 417.

11 Einarson A, Bailey B, Jung G *et al.* (1997) Prospective controlled study of hydroxyzine and cetirizine in pregnancy. *Ann Aller Asthma Immunol.* **78**(2): 183–6.

12 Pastuszak A, Schick B, D'Alimonte D *et al.* (1996) The safety of astemizole in pregnancy. *J Aller Clin Immunol.* **98**: 748–50.

13 Spangler JG, Kirk JK and Knudson MP (1994) Uses and safety of acyclovir in pregnancy. *J Fam Prac.* **38**(2): 186–91.

14 Boyd AS, Morris LF, Phillips CM *et al.* (1996) Psoriasis and pregnancy: hormone and immune system interaction. *Int J Dermatol.* **35**(3): 169–72.

15 Duley L (1999) Aspirin for preventing and treating pre-eclampsia. *BMJ.* **318**: 751–2.

16 van Schooten FJ (1996) Coal tar therapy: is it carcinogenic? *Drug Safety.* **15**(6): 374–7.

17 Lammer EJ, Hayes AM, Schunior A *et al.* (1987) Risk for major malformation among human fetuses exposed to isotretinoin (13-cis-retinoic acid). *Teratology.* **35**: 68A.

18 Gollnick HP (1996) Oral retinoids-efficacy and toxicity in psoriasis. *Br J Dermatol.* **135**(49): 6–17.

19 Marks R (1997) Clinical safety of tazarotene in the treatment of plaque psoriasis. *J Am Acad Dermatol.* **37**(3): S25–S32.

20 Chotiner HC (1985) Non-surgical management of ectopic pregnancy associated with severe hyperstimulation syndrome. *Obstet Gynecol.* **66**: 740–3.

21 Feldkamp M and Carey JC (1993) Clinical teratology counseling and consultation case report: low-dose methotrexate exposure in the early weeks of pregnancy. *Teratology.* **47**: 533–9.

22 Ostensen M and Ramsey-Goldman R (1998) Treatment of inflammatory rheumatic disorders in pregnancy. What are the safest treatment options? *Drug Safety.* **19**(5): 389–410.

23 British Medical Association and Royal Pharmaceutical Society (1998) *British National Formulary*, No. 36. Pharmaceutical Press, London.

24 Gunnarskog JG, Bengt Kallen AJ, Lindelof BG *et al.* (1993) Psoralen photochemotherapy (PUVA) and pregnancy. *Arch Dermatol.* **129**: 320–3.

25 Scroggins R (1999) Skin changes and diseases in pregnancy. In *Dermatology in General Medicine* (eds T Fitzpatrick, A Eiser, K Wolff *et al*). McGraw-Hill, New York.

26 Rothman KF and Pochi PE (1988) Use of oral and topical agents for acne in pregnancy. *J Am Acad Dermatol.* **16**(3): 431–43.

27 Czeizel AE and Rockenbauer M (1997) Teratogenic study of doxycycline. *Obstet Gynecol.* **89**: 524–8.

28 Keefe AM (1995) Adverse reactions profile: 12 retinoids. *Prescrib J.* **35**(2): 71–6.

29 Holmes SC, Bankowska U and Mackie RM (1998) The prescription of isotretinoin to women: is every precaution taken? *Br J Dermatol.* **138**(3): 450–5.

30 Jick H (1998) Retinoids and teratogenicity. *J Am Acad Dermatol.* **39**: S118–S122.

31 Jick SS, Terris BZ and Jick H (1993) First-trimester topical isotretinoin and congenital disorders. *Lancet.* **341**: 1181–2.

32 Shapiro L, Pastuszak A, Curto G *et al.* (1997) Safety of first-trimester exposure to topical tretinoin: prospective cohort study. *Lancet.* **350**: 1143–4.

33 Vaughan Jones SA and Black MM (1997) Skin problems in pregnancy. *Medicine.* **25**: 27–9.

34 Lawley T and Yancy K (1999) Skin changes and diseases in pregnancy. In *Dermatology in General Medicine* (eds T Fitzpatrick, A Eiser, K Wolff *et al.*). McGraw-Hill, New York.

CHAPTER SIXTEEN

Complementary/ alternative medicine during pregnancy

Edzard Ernst

Introduction

The use of complementary/alternative medicine (CAM) has become immensely popular. In the UK about 25% of the general population use some form of CAM.[1] In the USA this figure is 40%[2] and in Australia 50%.[3] The reasons for this demand are complex but one prominent motivator is clearly the hope of being cured without side-effects.

Side-effects are a particularly important issue for pregnant and lactating women. Potentially, they not only harm themselves but also their baby when choosing a treatment that is burdened with adverse effects. Thus one might assume that many such women will use CAM during pregnancy – which they assume is risk free. Surprisingly, there is little information on how many actually do. The only data available comes from Finland and was produced in the early 1990s.[4] This survey suggests that up to 14% of pregnant women use 'alternative drugs' (mostly herbal remedies and food supplements) at least once during their pregnancy. The figure for total CAM use is likely to be substantially higher.

In this chapter, those forms of CAM which are most likely to be used by pregnant and lactating women will be discussed briefly (it is impossible to mention them all – there are well over 100 different forms of CAM). In particular, the existing knowledge on their effectiveness and potential risks will be summarised.

Acupuncture

Acupuncture is an ancient Chinese therapy. It is based on the belief that two vital sources of 'energy' control our body – Yin and Yang. If they are 'in balance' we are healthy; when they are 'out of balance' we fall ill. Balance can then be restored by stimulating special points (acupuncture points) along the channels in which the energy flows, the meridians. Stimulation is usually given by sticking needles in these points, but other methods exist as well, e.g. pressure (acupressure), electricity (electroacupuncture) and heat (moxibustion).

These ancient Chinese concepts are based more on philosophy than on actual facts. For instance, no one has ever identified meridians or acupuncture points in a scientific manner. And so far no one has succeeded in measuring the vital 'energy' that forms the basis of the Chinese belief. Modern (medical or Western) acupuncturists have therefore tried to translate the old concepts into modern neurophysiology. They believe that acupuncture works through the stimulation of nerve endings and by releasing natural painkillers in the brain. There is increasingly good evidence for these concepts. Yet, at present, they remain hypothetical.

Today, both 'schools' of acupuncture exist side by side. Traditional Chinese acupuncturists will follow their old concepts of disease and diagnosis. Western acupuncturists are often physicians who use acupuncture mostly as an adjunct to orthodox medicines and insist on conventional diagnosis just as any other doctor would.

In pregnancy and lactation, acupuncture is promoted for three purposes in particular:

1   to alleviate the pain during childbirth
2   to ease back pain
3   to combat morning sickness.

Acupuncture for pain in childbirth

More and more women are in favour of 'natural' childbirth, hoping that this means a minimum of drugs. Therefore an effective drugless treatment against pain during childbirth would be very welcome. In fact, pains of all causes are the most frequent reason for using acupuncture today. The majority of (but not all) studies testing the effectiveness of acupuncture to alleviate pain suggest that it is effective.[5] The evidence on whether or not it helps specifically for pain in childbirth is not totally convincing but at least in part encouraging.

This means that, in the right circumstances, acupuncture is worth a try. Professional orthodox care should be on stand-by in case acupuncture fails, and the acupuncturist should be well trained and experienced. An ideal situation would be where the midwife also has expertise in acupuncture.

Acupuncture for back pain

Back pain is a very common problem in pregnancy and acupuncture can be an effective remedy. This has been shown in many controlled clinical trials.[6] Even though not all of them come to exactly the same conclusion, the evidence is, on balance, positive. Strictly speaking, this applies to 'normal' back pain and not to back pain of pregnancy. There are no trial data available for this particular indication. Yet there are no good reasons to assume that back pain during pregnancy responds fundamentally differently than 'normal' back pain. If a pregnant woman suffers from back pain, acupuncture is certainly worth a try.

Acupuncture for nausea/vomiting

Many women suffer from 'morning sickness' during early pregnancy. This is rarely a dangerous condition but it seriously impedes quality of life. What is worse, powerful drugs that stop nausea in other situations may be contraindicated in pregnancy. Therefore acupuncture and acupressure may be the solution.

The 'PC6' point is near the wrist on the inside of each arm. It can be stimulated by needling or, more easily, by applying pressure. Bands that are worn like bracelets are commercially available and will do the trick. The scientific evidence that this is effective is very convincing.[7] There are many good studies on the subject and they virtually all show that nausea and vomiting during pregnancy can be eased. They may not be totally eliminated but the symptoms will, in most cases, be much improved. The treatment must be carried out regularly.

Acupressure lends itself almost ideally to self-treatment and can be highly recommended to a patient suffering from 'morning sickness'.

Risk of acupuncture

The much promoted belief that acupuncture is entirely free of risks is certainly not true.[8] Pain and dizziness are common transient problems after acupuncture. Much more serious risks include infection through a non-sterile needle and injury of vital organs. Both types of complications should not occur in competent hands, but the sad truth is that they do still happen. The incidence is unknown but probably very low. The message here is to choose an acupuncturist carefully and ensure that he/she is highly competent.

Aromatherapy

Pregnancy can be a stressful time and relaxation greatly sought after. Many complementary therapies offer easy access to relaxation. Aromatherapy is one of these. Mood disturbances, nausea, stretch marks and pain are other relevant indications which aromatherapists feel confident in alleviating.

Aromatherapists use essential oils obtained from plants which they often apply to the skin through a gentle massaging action. The evidence for or against aromatherapy is shaky to say the least. What is more, its use in pregnancy or during lactation raises important safety issues. The often highly concentrated oils may be absorbed through the skin and enter the bloodstream. Thus they ought to be scrutinised in the same way as other drug treatment. In the absence of convincing safety data, aromatherapy oils cannot be recommended for pregnant or breastfeeding women.

Herbalism

It is tempting to use herbal remedies for a variety of conditions that arise during or after pregnancy, e.g.

- horsechestnut for venous insufficiency and swollen legs
- ginger for morning sickness
- St John's wort for postnatal depression.

For each of these (and many other) indications there is reasonably good clinical evidence to show that these treatments are effective for the respective conditions *outside* pregnancy. The usage of any oral drugs during pregnancy (and herbal remedies must be viewed as drugs in this context) is, however, a different matter. The prime concern must be to do no harm. In other words, we need conclusive evidence that herbs are risk free for the mother and fetus. For none of the above herbal remedies (or any other plant-based medicine) does such evidence exist. Thus herbal treatments should be viewed with caution and cannot be recommended during pregnancy or lactation.

Homoeopathy

Homoeopathy was developed 200 years ago by the German physician Samuel Hahnemann. It is based on the 'like-cures-like' principle which postulates that a remedy that causes certain symptoms in healthy individuals can be used to treat such symptoms when they present in a patient. The other major assumption of homoeopathy is that through 'potentising', that is, stepwise diluting and shaking a remedy, it will transmit 'energy' into the dilutant. Thus homoeopaths believe that even highly dilute remedies, which do not necessarily contain a single molecule of the initial substance, can still be clinically effective. This is the point which scientists find so deeply disturbing about homoeopathy. They simply insist: no molecule, no effect.

Notwithstanding this 200-year-old debate, the evidence from controlled clinical trials does, on balance, suggest that homoeopathic remedies are more than mere placebos.[9] Since highly dilute remedies are generally seen as totally free of side-effects, they might be considered for all sorts of ailments during pregnancy. Note that this applies only to highly dilute remedies!

Even though the hard evidence on whether homoeopathy is effective beyond a placebo effect is by no means compelling, one might take a 'liberal' view. If a patient has had good experience with homoeopathy she should carry on using it during pregnancy. In particular, it might be a wise choice for minor, non-threatening ailments. In cases of potentially serious diseases or complications of pregnancy, it is mandatory to consult a physician.

In summary, homeopathy appears to be safe in pregnancy but should not be relied upon to treat serious conditions as evidence regarding its effectiveness is limited.

Massage

As mentioned previously, massages can be very relaxing. In contrast to an aromatherapists, a massage therapist will rely on more forceful massage techniques which are usually directed at a specific, often musculoskeletal, pain. Back pain, for instance, may respond well to massage. Another ailment of pregnancy is stretch marks. There are certain massage techniques that have produced good results with this cosmetic problem.[10]

Massage can be safely used during pregnancy.

Reflexology

Reflexologists believe that the organs of the entire body are represented on the sole of the foot like a map of a geographical area. By palpating the foot they first diagnose the problem and subsequently treat it by massaging resistances and other abnormalities which they feel with their hands.

Even though there is no evidence that this concept is correct, reflexology may still do some good. The foot massage itself is relaxing and agreeable. If used as an adjunct to conventional care, it can do virtually no harm. Thus, if a pregnant woman feels better after reflexology there is little reason to advise her against it.

Spinal manipulation

Chiropractors and osteopaths believe that back pain and other conditions are caused by the misalignment of spinal motion segments. They normally take a careful history and detailed physical examination. Depending on the findings they may then manipulate the segment which is deemed to be affected. Treatments usually last about 20 minutes and most therapists would advocate a series of 6–12 sessions initially.

There is reasonably good, albeit not ultimately compelling, evidence to suggest that chiropractic or osteopathy can alleviate back pain.[11] The treatments are not entirely free of risk but there is no reason to fear that they could be damaging the fetus.

Complementary therapies to avoid

One may well take the view that, even in the absence of evidence for effectiveness, complementary therapies can help simply through making a pregnant patient feel better. This, however, applies only to treatments where the potential risks do not outweigh the potential benefits. There are several complementary treatments which, for this reason, should not be recommended during pregnancy. These include:

- aromatherapy (*see* above)
- blood letting
- cell therapy
- chelation therapy
- colonic irrigation
- extreme diets (e.g. Gerson diet, macrobiotics)
- food supplements in high doses
- herbalism (*see* above)
- rolfing.

Some final advice

None of the recommended complementary treatments should replace conventional care. However, some therapies can provide benefit when used wisely in conjunction with it. Women using complementary therapies should always tell their doctor and midwife which other therapies are being used.

A complementary therapist should be questioned about his/her:

- training
- experience
- indemnity cover.

Patients should be advised to avoid therapists who:

- try to alter their medications
- promise unreasonable things
- do not tell them how long they plan to treat and for what price
- speak badly about conventional medicine
- try to convince them to take dubious oral medications.

And finally, remember: if something sounds too good to be true, it probably is.

References

1 Fisher P and Ward A (1994) Complementary medicine in Europe. *BMJ.* **309**: 107–11.
2 Austin JA (1998) Why patients use alternative medicine. Results of a national study. *JAMA.* **279**: 1548-53.
3 MacLennan AH, Wilson DH and Taylor AW (1996) Prevalence and cost of alternative medicine in Australia. *Lancet.* **347**: 569–73.
4 Hemminki E, Mäntyranta T, Malin M *et al.* (1991) A survey on the use of alternative drugs during pregnancy. *Scand J Soc Med.* **19**(3): 199–204.
5 Ter Riet G, Kleijnen J and Knipschild P (1990) Acupuncture and chronic pain: a criterion-based meta-analysis. *J Clin Epidemiol.* **11**: 1191–9.
6 Ernst E and White AR (1998) Acupuncture for back pain: a meta-analysis of randomised controlled trials. *Arch Intern Med.* **158**: 2235–41.
7 Vickers AJ (1996) Can acupuncture have specific effects on health? A systematic review of acupuncture anti-emesis trials. *J Roy Soc Med.* **89**: 303–11.
8 Ernst E and White AR (1997) Life-threatening adverse reactions after acupuncture? A systematic review. *Pain.* **71**: 123–6.
9 Linde K, Claudius N, Ramirez G *et al.* (1997) Are the clinical effects of homoeopathy placebo effects? A meta-analysis of placebo-controlled trials. *Lancet.* **350**: 834–43.
10 Ernst E and Fialka V (1994) The clinical effectiveness of massage therapy: a critical review. *Forschende Komplement ärmedizin.* **1**: 226–32.
11 Ernst E and Assendelft WJJ (1998) Chiropractic for low back pain. We don't know whether it does more good than harm. *BMJ.* **317**: 160.

Recommended further reading

Cassileth BR (1998) *The Alternative Medicine Handbook.* WW Norton, New York.[1]
Ernst E (ed) (1996) *Complementary Medicine: an objective appraisal.* Butterworth, Oxford.[2]
Newall CA, Anderson LA and Phillipson JD (1996) *Herbal Medicines: a guide for healthcare professionals*, pp. 250–2. The Pharmaceutical Press, London.[2]
Rowlands B (1997) *The Which? Guide to Complementary Medicine.* Consumers' Association, London.[1]
Fugh-Berman A (1996) *Alternative Medicine: what works.* Odonian Press, Tucson, Arizona.[1]
Schulz V, Hänsel R and Tyler VE (1997) *Rational Phytotherapy.* Springer, Berlin.[2]

[1] Primarily written for a lay readership.
[2] Primarily written for a professional readership.

CHAPTER SEVENTEEN

Social drugs

Simon Wills

Introduction

Alcohol, tobacco and caffeine are often referred to as so-called 'social drugs'. The effects of these agents on human pregnancy outcome and breastfeeding have been studied quite extensively.

Alcohol

A large number of published studies attest to the harmful effects of alcohol during human pregnancy, and a number of reviews have been published.[1–4] The precise effects of maternal drinking are hard to evaluate because it is almost impossible to separate the effects of alcohol from confounding factors such as smoking, socio-economic status, ethnicity and diet.[5–10] A low-level alcohol consumption during pregnancy, e.g. one unit per day, has not been proven to adversely affect the infant. Many clinicians take the line of most caution, recommending abstention from alcohol during pregnancy. This is needlessly draconian. Pregnant women who drink less than 10 units per week are not at risk of giving birth to a damaged baby.[11] The research is consistent in finding no evidence of fetal harm at these levels, providing that the drinking is spread over several days and not all drunk at once.[11]

Frequent drinkers are defined as women who drink more than 10 units per week but are not alcohol dependent. These women may be at risk of giving birth to a baby with a number of individual abnormalities – fetal alcohol effects (FAE). The effects include cardiac, urogenital and neuro-anatomical anomalies as well as attention deficit disorders. The association between frequent drinking and these abnormalities remains controversial.[11]

The fetal alcohol syndrome (FAS) occurs in babies born to women who are dependent on alcohol. These women are heavy drinkers who rely on alcohol and are unable to control the amount they drink. They are likely to consume at least six units of alcohol every day.[12–16] The risk ranges from one in 50 to one in four, depending on factors such as race and socio-economic status. Black women seem to be at much greater risk than other women.[17,18] In general, the heaviest drinkers seem to be delivered of the most badly affected infants. The three cardinal features of FAS are facial anomalies, CNS dysfunction and pre- and postnatal growth deficiency. Babies with FAS have at least one feature in each of these categories. A more detailed list is given in Box 17.1. Congenital heart disease may be associated with FAS, especially ventricular septal defects. Various other abnormalities have also been linked with the syndrome, including limb defects, urogenital deformities and liver damage but there is insufficient evidence to establish a true association. The incidence of FAS in the West is probably between one and six cases per 3000 live births.

Box 17.1: Features of fetal alcohol syndrome

- Facial abnormalities: thin upper lip, elongated/flat mid-face, short palpebral fissures, microphthalmia, indistinct philtrum, short upturned nose, small jaw, other jaw deformities, low-set ears
- CNS defects: microcephaly, neurological impairment, delayed development, neurobehavioural anomalies, brain abnormalities
- Growth retardation: prenatal, postnatal, or both

It is not clear how harmful a single episode of heavy drinking in pregnancy may be. Women who are concerned about occasional excessive drinking before being aware of the pregnancy should be advised that the risk is likely to be small.[11] The evidence of an association between alcohol consumption and miscarriage is conflicting and inconclusive.[19–23] Moderate to heavy alcohol intake during pregnancy is associated with an increased risk of spontaneous abortions and stillbirths. Although prematurity is linked to FAS, it has not been shown to occur outside this setting. Chronic heavy drinking in late pregnancy can cause withdrawal reactions in some babies. These are characterised by tremors, apnoea, cyanosis, hypertonia, irritability, abdominal distension, and even convulsions. In general the symptoms only last a few days.

Although it is difficult to generalise, babies affected by FAS may continue to be affected by their condition into childhood.[24,25] During early school years they may still exhibit growth retardation, intellectual deficits and behavioural disorders. The facial features tend to disappear in adult life, although the long philtrum and microcephaly are the most persistent. The persistence of any neurobehavioural deficit in children exposed to alcohol, but who do not suffer from FAS, has not been adequately explored.

Taking time in early pregnancy with the relatively few women who drink heavily and then providing relevant information helps some to reduce their consumption. In non-pregnant subjects, a brief 15–20 minute intervention of this kind has been shown to be just as effective as more expensive specialist treatments. It results in a reduction in alcohol consumption of 10% in alcohol-dependent individuals.

Pregnant women should be advised that drinking less than 10 units of alcohol a week is unlikely to harm their baby. Any such drinking should be spread out over the week. GPs and midwives should make time available to offer frequent drinkers and alcohol-dependent women counselling and sensitive advice. Healthy women who have drunk to the point of drunkenness once or twice in early pregnancy can be reassured that there is a minimal risk of their baby being harmed.

Breastfeeding

Alcohol enters breast milk, reaching a concentration that approximates to that in the maternal plasma. After suckling it is absorbed into the baby's circulation. Neonates and infants have disproportionately reduced amounts of alcohol dehydrogenase compared to adults and so alcohol clearance is slow.

Although one case of apparent 'drunkenness' in an infant exposed to alcohol via breast milk was described in 1937, no similar cases have been reported in the literature.[26] An isolated case report described the development of Cushing's syndrome in an infant who was breast-fed by a woman who habitually drank large amounts of alcohol. When maternal alcohol intake ceased, the signs of Cushing's syndrome slowly resolved.[27]

Limited research has investigated the potential long-term effects upon the infant of exposure to alcohol via breast milk. In one study in Mexico, growth was measured in 32 breast-fed babies whose mothers consumed up to 2 litres of pulque (3% alcohol) per day.[28] There was no difference in postnatal growth compared to controls. Mental development of the infants was not assessed. Another study, of middle-class American women who drank during breastfeeding, revealed that there was a dose-dependent impairment of psychomotor development of the infant at one year of age.[29] Unfortunately, no follow-up study of these children has been published. Similar studies are needed to verify whether this is a true effect of alcohol.

Alcohol impairs the ejection of milk from the breast in a dose-dependent way, by inhibiting the release of oxytocin.[30] Regular high intake of alcohol may thus suppress milk supply. However, even small amounts of alcohol may reduce the amount of milk consumed by suckling infants by up to a quarter. The reasons for this are unclear.[31]

Since the effects of alcohol upon the infant are not clear, women may wish to restrict their intake while breastfeeding. If alcohol is consumed, it should be shortly after feeding and some time before the next feed is due. The rate of alcohol clearance from the body is dose-dependent, and as women clear more slowly than men, avoiding breastfeeding for two hours for each unit of alcohol consumed, minimises infant exposure.

Caffeine

Caffeine may decrease female fertility. Initial studies investigating the time to conception in women wishing to become pregnant revealed a greater latency in women consuming caffeine.[32–34] These relatively small studies appeared to show a dose-related effect with even small amounts of caffeine having an effect. A more recent study suggested a significant effect on female fertility only at very high levels of consumption (i.e. above 500 mg daily),[35] and that the effect was potentiated by cigarette smoking. However, in the largest study to date, involving 10 886 women, no relationship could be found between caffeine intake and fertility, except in a group of women who drank in excess of eight cups of coffee a day and who also smoked tobacco.[36]

A large number of studies have shown that caffeine is neither teratogenic nor linked to premature delivery. However, caffeine has been associated with other adverse pregnancy outcomes – specifically, decreased neonatal birth weight and an increased risk of spontaneous abortion. Unfortunately, many early studies failed to take account of the possible effects of tobacco smoking and/or alcohol intake on the measured parameters. Consequently, it is impossible to assess their significance.

Recent studies of the effects of caffeine upon birth weight have provided conflicting results, including: no adverse effects;[37] no significant effect except in smokers with high caffeine intake;[38] no adverse effects on fetal weight unless dose exceeds 70 mg daily;[39] unless dose exceeds 300 mg daily;[40] or a dose-related effect with some adverse effects at all levels of consumption.[41] In the face of this conflicting data it would seem wise to suggest that pregnant women limit their caffeine intake until further studies provide a consensus view on the likelihood of any ill effects. During the second and third trimesters the ability to metabolise caffeine is reduced, and caffeine blood levels may rise even though intake remains stable. This could potentiate any adverse effects upon fetal development.

Many studies have attempted to assess the role of caffeine in triggering spontaneous abortion. Again, most of the earlier studies fail to take account of the impact of maternal smoking, alcohol, drugs or obstetric history. More recent research has shown either a very weak link or no link.[40,42,43] More carefully designed research is needed to clarify the situation.

While most studies have failed to find adverse effects in neonates exposed to caffeine *in utero*, one study identified withdrawal effects in babies exposed to particularly high concentrations (an estimated average of 863 mg caffeine per day). The eight infants suffered from symptoms such as irritability, jitteriness and vomiting. Caffeine was detected in the plasma of six of them.[44] In another study, 16 babies exposed to at least 500 mg caffeine per day were compared to babies exposed to a maximum of 250 mg per day. The high exposure babies exhibited a markedly increased incidence of tremors, tachyarrhythmias, tachypnoea and premature atrial contractions.[45]

Breastfeeding

Caffeine passes into breast milk. The extent of such transfer has been the subject of numerous studies, all of which confirm that although caffeine readily passes into milk it does not accumulate.[46–51] The concentration in milk is not known to exceed 90% of maternal plasma or saliva levels. Where neonatal plasma or urine concentrations of caffeine have been measured after ingestion of milk from mothers who consumed caffeine, the levels have been extremely low and often undetectable.[46–48] Few adverse effects have been noted in infants given milk containing caffeine, and when these have occurred they have been mild and reversible, e.g. irritability and sleeplessness. Serious effects that might be anticipated with high plasma levels, such as tachycardia, convulsions and vomiting, have not been described.

Caffeine is used therapeutically to treat neonatal respiratory problems such as apnoea. The doses given intravenously to the neonate are far greater than those arising from exposure to caffeine-laden breast milk, and without notable adverse effect. Doses used can be in excess of 10 mg/kg body weight. However, neonates and infants do metabolise caffeine much more slowly than adults – the half-life being an average of 100 hours in the newborn, and up to 230 hours in the premature neonate, compared to five hours in adults. This does lead to the possibility of accumulation.

The consumption of caffeinated foods and beverages is not contraindicated during breastfeeding. But if mothers notice any of the above adverse effects in the breast-fed infant, their caffeine consumption should be reduced.

Tobacco

Cigarette smoking in pregnancy has been studied very extensively, and the reader is referred to a number of excellent reviews.[52–56] When smoked, cigarettes release a number of chemicals including nicotine, carbon monoxide, tar and cyanide. Many, if not all, of the associated adverse pregnancy outcomes may be simply the result of fetal hypoxia.

Intra-uterine growth retardation (IUGR) and decreased birth weight have been strongly and consistently linked with smoking in pregnancy. Adverse effects upon growth are probably dose-related, but do not seem to occur if women stop smoking before the end of the first trimester. Unfortunately, passive smoking also leads to adverse effects on growth.

The rate of spontaneous abortion, stillbirth and neonatal death is markedly increased in women who smoke. However, the association between premature delivery and smoking is less clear. Some studies suggest that any effect of smoking is augmented by caffeine. Smoking also incurs a significantly increased risk of abruptio placentae, placenta previa and premature membrane rupture.

Exposure to tobacco smoke is not strongly associated with an increased incidence of congenital malformations. No major fetal abnormalities have been conclusively linked to tobacco. Some studies report a small overall increased risk of all congenital abnormalities, but many do not. However, high levels of fetal exposure during pregnancy have been shown to increase the risk of impaired physical development, mental retardation, and behavioural anomalies in childhood.

Box 17.2: Effects of tobacco smoking in pregnancy

Increased risk of:

- intrauterine growth retardation
- reduced birth weight
- spontaneous abortion
- stillbirth
- neonatal death
- abruptio placenta, placenta praevia and premature membrane rupture.

Breastfeeding

Nicotine and its main metabolite, cotinine, readily pass into breast milk and both can be detected in the serum of the breast-fed infant.[57–61] The breast milk of smokers contains higher concentrations of cadmium than non-smokers, but the amount present is much less than the maximum acceptable intake from normal diet.[62] Apart from this, the passage of other constituents of tobacco smoke into breast milk has not been studied. Apart from the tobacco constituents that enter breast milk, it should be noted that babies are directly exposed to tobacco smoke when people smoke near to them – so-called 'passive smoking'. Hence plasma from bottle-fed babies whose mothers smoke also contains nicotine, albeit in smaller amounts.[58,59]

The American Academy of Pediatrics lists a variety of possible adverse effects in infants exposed to nicotine-laden breast milk.[63] These include vomiting, diarrhoea, tachycardia and restlessness. These symptoms all seem to be based on a single case report from 1937[26] and have not been described in the literature since. However, it is documented that babies exposed to nicotine in breast milk may develop colic.[60,64] Babies exposed to passive smoking are also more susceptible to respiratory tract infections.[61,65] In adults, passive smoking is known to be carcinogenic. It has been suggested that passive smoking by babies may be associated with sudden infant death syndrome (SIDS).

It is recognised that women who smoke are less likely to breastfeed and that in those who do the duration of breastfeeding tends to be shorter than in non-smokers.[58,66] This has been linked with nicotine-induced reduction in maternal prolactin levels,[67,68] although more recently it has been suggested that the higher levels of somatostatin in smokers may be responsible for early weaning.[69]

In summary:

- nicotine passes into breast milk and can cause colic in the infant
- smoking may prevent breastfeeding or limit its duration
- passive smoking is carcinogenic and is associated with an increased risk of respiratory tract infection in the infant, and may also be linked to SIDS
- breastfeeding mothers should minimise tobacco smoking and avoid smoking in the vicinity of infants
- smoking just after breastfeeding will reduce nicotine exposure through milk, since the half-life in adults is about two hours.

Table 17.1: Social drugs in pregnancy

Drug	Effects on fetus	Neonatal withdrawal reported
Alcohol	Fetal Alcohol Syndrome (facial dysmorphism, CNS defect and reduced growth) – probably dose-related	+
Caffeine	Large doses possibly decrease maternal fertility Probably does not cause malformations	+
Tobacco	Reduced growth, increased spontaneous abortions, abruptions, stillbirths and neonatal deaths	–

Table 17.2: Summary of effects on infant of social drugs in breastfeeding women

General advice:	1	Avoid breastfeeding while maternal plasma levels are still high
	2	Avoid exposing baby to peak milk levels of drug, by taking drug after a breastfeed
	3	Monitor baby for adverse effects

Drug	Importance of avoiding in breastfeeding	Can impair breastfeeding	Important neonatal clearance deficit	Effects upon infant
Alcohol	+	Yes	Yes	Lack of convincing evidence for harm at low intake
Caffeine	–	No	Yes	Possible irritability or sleeplessness
Tobacco	–	Yes	No	Neonatal colic described – avoid exposing infant to passive smoking

References

1 Young NK (1997) Effects of alcohol and other drugs on children. *J Psychoactive Drugs.* **29**: 23–42.
2 Tuormaa TE (1996) The adverse effects of alcohol on reproduction. *J Nutritional Med.* **6**: 379–91.
3 Coles CD (1993) Impact of prenatal alcohol exposure on the newborn and the child. *Clin Obs Gynecol.* **36**: 255–66.
4 National Institute on Alcohol Abuse and Alcoholism (1991) Fetal alcohol syndrome. *Alcohol Alert.* **13**: 1–4.
5 Walpole I, Zubrick S and Pontre J (1989) Confronting variables in studying the effects of maternal alcohol consumption before and during pregnancy. *J Epidem Comm Health.* **43**(2): 153–61.
6 Rurak DW (1992) Fetal behavioural states: pathological alterations with drug/alcohol abuse. *Semin Prenatal.* **16**(4): 239–51.
7 Glantz JC and Woods JR (1993) Cocaine, heroin and phencyclidine: obstetric perspectives. *Clin Obstet Gynecol.* **36**(2): 279–301.
8 Stephens CJ (1985) Alcohol consumption during pregnancy among southern city women. *Drug Alcoh Depend.* **16**.
9 Abel EL and Sokol RJ (1987) Incidence of fetal alcohol syndrome and economic impact of FAS-related anomalies. *Drug Alcoh Depend.* **19**: 51–70.
10 Zambrana RE, Hernandez M, Dunkel-Schetter C *et al.* (1991) Ethnic differences in the substance use patterns of low-income pregnant women. *Fam Comm Health.* **13**(4): 1–11.
11 Plant M, Sullivan FM *et al.* (1994) Alcohol and pregnancy. In PM Verschuren (ed) *Health Issues Related to Alcohol Consumption.* Cardiff Academic Press, Cardiff.
12 Sokol RJ, Miller SI, Debanne S *et al.* (1981) The Cleveland NIAAA prospective alcohol in pregnancy study: the first year. *Neurobehav Toxicol Teratol.* **3**(2): 203–9.

13 Streissguth AP, Martin DC, Martin JC *et al.* (1981) The Seattle longitudinal prospective study on alcohol and pregnancy. *Neurobehav Toxicol Teratol.* **3**(2): 223–33.

14 Kuzma JW and Kissinger DG (1981) Patterns of alcohol and cigarette use in pregnancy. *Neurobehav Toxicol Teratol.* **3**(2): 211–21.

15 Rosett HL, Weiner L, Lee A *et al.* (1983) Patterns of alcohol consumption and fetal development. *Obstet Gynecol.* **61**(5): 539–46.

16 Weiner L, Rosett HL, Edelin KC *et al.* (1983) Alcohol consumption by pregnant women. *Obstet Gynecol.* **61**(1): 6–12.

17 Plant M, Sullivan FM *et al.* (1994) Alcohol and pregnancy. In PM Verschuren (ed) *Health Issues Related to Alcohol Consumption.* Cardiff Academic Press, Cardiff, pp 245–62.

18 Sonderegger TB (1992) *Perinatal Substance Abuse: research findings and clinical implications.* Johns Hopkins University Press, Baltimore.

19 Harlap S and Shiono PH (1980) Alcohol, smoking and incidence of spontaneous abortions in the first and second trimester. *Lancet.* **26 July**: 173–6.

20 Russell M and Skinner JB (1988) Early measures of maternal alcohol misuse as predictors of adverse pregnancy outcomes. *Alcoh Clin Exp Res.* **12**(6): 824–30.

21 Armstrong BG, McDonald AD and Sloan M (1992) Cigarette, alcohol and coffee consumption and spontaneous abortion. *Am J Pub Health.* **82**(1): 85–7.

22 Windham GC, Fenster L and Swan SH (1992) Moderate maternal and paternal alcohol consumption and the risk of spontaneous abortion. *Epidemiol.* **3**(4): 364–70.

23 Halmesmaki E, Valimaki M, Roine R *et al.* (1989) Maternal and paternal alcohol consumption and miscarriage. *Br J Obstet Gynaecol.* **96**(2): 188–91.

24 Eckardt MJ, File SE, Gessa GL *et al.* (1998) Effects of moderate alcohol consumption on the central nervous system. *Alcoh Clin Exp Res.* **22**(5): 998–1040.

25 Aronson M and Hagberg B (1998) Neuropsychological disorders in children exposed to alcohol during pregnancy: a follow-up study of 24 children born to alcoholic mothers in Goteborg, Sweden. *Alcoh Clin Exp Res.* **22**(2): 321–4.

26 Bisdom W (1937) Alcohol and nicotine poisoning in nurslings. *J Am Med Assoc.* **109**: 178.

27 Binkiewicz A, Robinson MJ and Senior B (1978) Pseudo-Cushing syndrome caused by alcohol in breast milk. *J Pediatr.* **93**: 965–7.

28 Flores-Huerta S, Hernandez-Montes H, Argote RM and Villalpando S (1992) Effects of ethanol consumption during pregnancy and lactation on the outcome and postnatal growth of the offspring. *Ann Nutrition Metabolism.* **36**: 121–8.

29 Little RE, Anderson KW and Ervin CH *et al.* (1989) Maternal alcohol use during breast-feeding and infant mental and motor development at one year. *New Engl J Med.* **321**: 425–30.

30 Cobo E (1973) Effect of different doses of ethanol on the milk-ejecting reflex in lactating women. *Am J Obs Gyn.* **115**: 817–21.

31 Mennella JA and Beauchamp GK (1991) The transfer of alcohol to human milk: effects on flavor and the infant's behavior. *New Engl J Med.* **325**: 981–5.

32 Wilcox A, Weinberg C and Baird D (1988) Caffeinated beverages and decreased fertility. *Lancet.* **2**: 1453–6.

33 Christianson RE, Oechsli FW and van den Berg BJ (1989) Caffeinated beverages and decreased fertility. *Lancet.* **1**: 378.

34 Williams MA, Monson RR, Goldman MB *et al.* (1990) Coffee and delayed conception. *Lancet.* **335**: 1603.

35   Bolumar F, Olsen J, Rebagliato M *et al.* (1997) Caffeine intake and delayed conception: a European multicenter study on infertility and sub-fecundity. *Am J Epidemiol.* **145**: 324–34.

36   Olsen J (1991) Cigarette smoking, tea and coffee drinking and subfecundity. *Am J Epidemiol.* **133**: 734–9.

37   Shu XO, Hatch MC, Mills J *et al.* (1995) Maternal smoking, alcohol drinking, caffeine consumption and fetal growth: results from a prospective study. *Epidemiol.* **6**: 115–20.

38   Cook DG, Peacock JL, Feyeraband C *et al.* (1996) Relation of caffeine intake and blood caffeine concentrations during pregnancy to fetal growth: prospective population based study, *BMJ.* **313**: 1358–62.

39   Vlajinac HD, Petrovic RR, Marinkovic JM *et al.* (1997) Effect of caffeine intake during pregnancy on birth weight. *Am J Epidemiol.* **145**: 335–8.

40   Fenster L, Eskenazi B, Windham GC and Swan SH (1991) Caffeine consumption during pregnancy and fetal growth. *Am J Pub Health.* **81**: 458–61.

41   Martin TR and Bracken MB (1987) The association between low birth weight and caffeine consumption during pregnancy. *Am J Epidemiol.* **126**: 813–21.

42   Olsen J, Overvad K and Frische G (1991) Coffee consumption, birth weight and reproductive failures. *Epidemiol.* **3**: 370–4.

43   Armstrong BG, McDonald AD and Sloan M (1992) Cigarette, alcohol and coffee consumption and spontaneous abortion. *Am J Pub Health.* **82**: 85–7.

44   McGowan JD, Altman RE and Kanto WP (1988) Neonatal withdrawal symptoms after chronic maternal ingestion of caffeine. *South Med J.* **81**: 1092–4.

45   Hadeed A and Siegel S (1993) Newborn cardiac arrhythmias associated with maternal caffeine use during pregnancy. *Clin Ped.* **32**: 45–7.

46   Ryu JE (1985) Caffeine in human milk and in serum of breast-fed infants. *Dev Pharmacol Ther.* **8**: 329–37.

47   Ryu JE (1985) Effect of maternal caffeine consumption on heart rate and sleep time of breast-fed infants, *Dev Pharmacol Ther.* **8**: 355–63.

48   Hildebrandt R and Gundert-Remy U (1983) *Ped Pharmacol.* **3**: 237–44.

49   Stavchansky S, Combs A, Sagraves R *et al.* (1988) Pharmacokinetics of caffeine in breast milk and plasma after single oral administration of caffeine to lactating mothers. *Biopharmaceutics Drug Disposition.* **9**: 285–99.

50   Berlin Jr CM, Denson HM, Daniel C and Ward RM (1984) Disposition of dietary caffeine in milk, saliva and plasma of lactating women. *Pediatrics.* **73**: 59–63.

51   Nehlig A and Debry G (1994) Consequences on the newborn of chronic maternal consumption of coffee during gestation and lactation: a review. *Am Coll Nutrition.* **13**: 6–21.

52   Fried PA (1993) Prenatal exposure to tobacco and marijuana: effects during pregnancy, infancy and early childhood. *Clin Obs Gynecol.* **36**: 319–37.

53   Folb PI and Dukes MN (1990) Cigarette smoking. In PI Folb and MN Dukes (eds) *Drug Safety in Pregnancy.* Elsevier Science, Oxford.

54   Stillman RJ, Rosenberg MJ and Sachs BP (1986) Smoking and reproduction. *Fertil Steril.* **46**: 545–66.

55   Freidman JM and Polifka JE (1994) Cigarette smoking (tobacco). In JM Friedman and JE Polifka (eds) *Teratogenic Effects of Drugs: a resource for clinicians.* Johns Hopkins, Baltimore.

56   Bell GL and Lau K (1995) Perinatal and neonatal issues of substance abuse. *Ped Clin N America.* **42**: 261–81.

57   Ferguson BB, Wilson DJ and Schaffner W (1976) Determination of nicotine concentrations in human milk. *Am J Dis Child.* **130**: 837–9.

58   Schwartz-Bickenbach D, Schulte-Holbein B, Abt S *et al.* (1987) Smoking and passive smoking during pregnancy and early infancy: effects on birth weight, lactation period, and cotinine concentrations in mother's milk and infant's urine. *Toxicol Lett.* **35**: 73–81.

59   Labrecque M, Marcoux S, Weber J-P *et al.* (1989) Feeding and urine cotinine values in babies whose mothers smoke. *Pediatrics.* **83**: 93–7.

60   Matheson I and Rivrud GN (1989) The effect of smoking on lactation and infantile colic. *J Am Med Assoc.* **261**: 42–3.

61   Schulte-Hobein B, Schwartz-Bickenbach D, Abt S *et al.* (1992) Cigarette smoke exposure and development of infants throughout the first year of life: influence of passive smoking and nursing on cotinine levels in breast milk and infant's urine. *Acta Paediatrica.* **81**: 550–7.

62   Raisch B, Luck W and Nau H (1987) Cadmium concentrations in milk and blood of smoking mothers. *Toxicol Lett.* **36**: 147–52.

63   Committee on Drugs (1994) The transfer of drugs and other chemicals into human milk. *Pediatrics.* **93**: 137–50.

64   Said G, Patois E and Lellouch J (1984) Infantile colic and parental smoking. *BMJ.* **289**: 660.

65   Hakansson A and Cars H (1991) Maternal cigarette smoking, breastfeeding and respiratory tract infections in infancy: a matched pairs study. *Scand J Prim Health Care.* **9**: 115–19.

66   Whichelow MJ and King BE (1979) Breast feeding and smoking. *Arch Dis Child.* **54**: 240–5.

67   Berta L, Frairia R, Fortuanti N *et al.* (1992) Smoking effects on the hormonal balance of fertile women. *Hormone Res.* **37**: 45–8.

68   Phil GS, Albala C, Yanez M *et al.* (1995) Smoking effects on prolactin at the end of pregnancy. *Nutrition Res.* **15**: 1599–604.

69   Widstrom A-M, Werner S, Mathieson A-S *et al.* (1991) Somatostatin levels in plasma in non-smoking and smoking breastfeeding women. *Acta Paed Scand.* **80**: 13–21.

CHAPTER EIGHTEEN

Street drugs

Simon Wills

Introduction

It is difficult to evaluate all the published data concerning drugs of abuse in human pregnancy and breastfeeding. While some areas have been studied in depth (e.g. cocaine in pregnancy), most have not been investigated with any degree of thoroughness. Moreover, the data are frequently lacking in quality as well as quantity. Authors often fail to take account of confounding variables such as socioeconomic status or the use of other pharmacologically active substances when investigating the effects of one particular drug. Many of the older studies tend to omit vital details on dose of drug, frequency of use and trimester(s) of exposure. The data on drugs in breastfeeding are particularly poor, and there are similarly little data on long-term effects of *in utero* exposure. Where the literature approaches a consensus, the details available have been simply summarised without referral to individual papers. Where there are limited or conflicting data, the information available has been evaluated in the hope of offering the most useful advice.

Amphetamine and Ecstasy

A retrospective study of 184 infants with congenital heart disease revealed an increased rate of therapeutic amphetamine use by their mothers during pregnancy, compared to controls.[1] Another study of 119 first-trimester exposures to amphetamines revealed a neonatal malformation rate of 137 per 1000 live births, compared to 20–30 per 1000 in the non-exposed general population.[2] The incidence of congenital heart disease was raised from 5–10 per 1000, to 25 cases per 1000. Interestingly, this study included 92 cases of Ecstasy use during pregnancy. A number of other studies of amphetamine and its derivatives have failed to find an association with malformations.[3–6] In total, these studies include over 3000 pregnancies.

Possible links with oral clefts and neonatal biliary atresia have been suggested due to amphetamine exposure *in utero*.[4,7] However, the numbers involved in these studies are too small for accurate interpretation and no other studies have verified these findings.

Fetal growth retardation, reduced body weight, prematurity and reduced neonatal head circumference may all be more common in babies born to those who abuse amphetamines.[5,8–10] These problems are also common to many babies born to women who abuse other street drugs or alcohol during pregnancy, but the studies involving street amphetamines are small and often yield conflicting or barely significant results. These complications have not been reported with therapeutic amphetamine exposure, suggesting that maternal lifestyle may be an important determinant.

Withdrawal reactions have been reported in some neonates delivered of amphetamine abusers. Reactions include abnormal sleep patterns, tremor, poor feeding, hypertonia, high pitched cry, vomiting, sneezing and excessive sucking.[8,11] However, some studies have failed to identify any neonatal withdrawal symptoms.[5]

Eriksson and colleagues in Sweden followed a group of 65 amphetamine exposed fetuses from birth to 10 years of age. Compared to unexposed children, boys were not significantly shorter or lighter at birth, one year, or four years of age, but a significant difference was apparent at age eight years. For exposed girls, the reverse was true – significantly lighter and shorter at birth, one year and four years, but not at aged eight.[12] At aged 10, eight of them (12%) attended a school class one year below that of their biological age, compared to the national average of about 5%. At ages four and eight, there was an increased incidence of aggression.[13]

The suspected serotonergic neurotoxic effects of Ecstasy in the CNS give additional cause for concern.[14]

Breastfeeding

Only one case history of maternal use of amphetamine during breastfeeding has been documented.[15] A woman with narcolepsy took dexamphetamine (5 mg, four times daily) while breastfeeding. Amphetamine appeared to concentrate in breast milk – on the tenth post-partum day, the concentration in milk was three times higher than that in maternal plasma, and by day 42 it was seven times greater. Neonatal plasma levels were not measured and the baby appeared to suffer no ill effects.

An unpublished study of 103 women who took amphetamines while breastfeeding was cited in 1973 and no adverse effects were reported in infants.[16] However, this study has never been published and its validity cannot be relied upon.

In pregnant women, amphetamine reduces plasma prolactin levels in a dose-dependent way.[17,18] It is therefore possible that regular high-dose amphetamine might impair milk production. Because of the paucity of data available it would be advisable for regular amphetamine users not to breastfeed. When administered directly to infants, amphetamines can cause either stimulation or sedation and mothers who choose to take amphetamines and breastfeed should monitor their babies for either reaction. If side effects do occur they could worsen with time, as the drug may accumulate in milk.

There are no data on the pharmacokinetics of Ecstasy in breastfeeding. However, given their chemical and structural similarity, Ecstasy would be expected to behave in a similar manner to amphetamine, and it too should be avoided by breastfeeding mothers. The long-term effects of the potential CNS neurotoxic effects of Ecstasy on the neonate are unknown.[14]

Anabolic steroids

Pregnancy

Anabolic steroid abuse usually reduces female fertility, and no pregnancies in abusers have been described in the literature. However, since high doses of androgenic drugs normally cause amenorrhoea, women taking these drugs may not realise if they ovulate and become pregnant. This could lead to a considerable duration of inadvertent exposure during early pregnancy.

Information is available on the use of therapeutic doses of testosterone and methyltestosterone,[19] and danazol during human pregnancy.[20–24] All three of these androgenic drugs can cause virilisation of the female fetus, as can certain progestogens with androgenic properties. These reactions have included: labial fusion, clitoral enlargement, development of a small phallus, ambiguous genitalia, and increased neonatal serum testosterone levels. Development of the external genitalia is complete by the end of the first trimester, so major physical changes require first-trimester exposure to androgens. Exposure after the first trimester tends to result only in an enlarged clitoris. However, in all published cases these problems resolved spontaneously or after minor surgery. Due to lack of tissue differentiation, exposure before the eighth week of pregnancy is unlikely to have harmful effects.

There are limited data on the subsequent physical, emotional or sexual development of these babies. Three papers describe the development to puberty and beyond of 14 girls who were exposed to virilising drugs *in utero* and suffered genital anomalies. All menstruated normally.[25–27] By the time of reporting, two of the women had successfully conceived. Adverse effects of androgenic drugs in male fetuses have not been described.

Breastfeeding

There are no published studies of anabolic steroid abuse by breastfeeding women. It is also not known whether anabolic steroids penetrate human breast milk. Chemically, these drugs are very lipophilic, but they are also highly protein bound and this may limit milk penetration.

A notable adverse effect of anabolic steroid abuse in women is reduction in breast size – an effect which is often irreversible. This may inhibit lactation in women who have used these drugs extensively before conception. Furthermore, anabolic steroids have been used therapeutically, with varying success, to suppress lactation. Higher doses have been reasonably successful[28–30] while smaller doses were ineffective.[31,32] Consequently women who start to take anabolic steroids while breastfeeding, or who resume an occasional habit, may find that lactation abruptly ceases. Anabolic steroids are believed to inhibit the action of prolactin but not its release. If a woman taking anabolic steroids does successfully breastfeed there may be some risk of virilisation of female babies.

Cannabis

Pregnancy

Many studies have investigated the effects of cannabis on human pregnancy outcomes, and several reviews have been published.[33–37] When demographic differences and other confounding variables are taken into account, none of them show cannabis to be teratogenic. Case reports of fetal deformities show no particular pattern – cannabis use is common and any association is thought to be spurious.

It has been suggested that cannabis use during pregnancy may be associated with delayed development of the central nervous system.[37] This is based on observations, from several studies, that cannabis can cause unusual neonatal behaviour such as persistent tremors and exaggerated startles, atypical sleep cycles, high pitched crying, and reduced visual habituation. However, such a link must remain speculative until more definitive studies have been performed.

One study of 1690 pregnancies suggested a five fold increased risk of fetal alcohol syndrome in women who drank small amounts of alcohol during pregnancy but who also smoked cannabis.[38] However, the number of pregnancies in this category was relatively few and this has not been confirmed in larger studies.

Most studies have not linked cannabis use to low birth weight. The validity of the small number of studies that suggest such a link is doubtful due to poor study design, inconsistent results, or inadequate control for confounding variables. There is insufficient information to ascertain whether fetal exposure has any meaningful ill effects upon behavioural or cognitive development during childhood.

In 1989, an epidemiological study of 204 children with acute non-lymphoblastic leukaemia, revealed that 10 of them had been exposed to cannabis *in utero*.[39] In the matched control group of 203 children, only one mother had used a street drug during pregnancy. This suggested that cannabis exposure during uterine development may be linked to a 10-fold increased risk of developing this form of leukaemia. Interviews with the parents of 322 young patients with rhabdomyosarcoma, revealed that maternal use of cannabis during the year before delivery was associated with a three-fold increased risk of offspring developing the cancer[40] Paternal use of cannabis increased the risk by two fold. Both of these studies need to be repeated before any firm conclusions can be drawn.

Breastfeeding

Cannabis contains a range of pharmacologically active compounds, but the principal psychoactive constituent is delta-9-tetrahydrocannabinol (THC). The 60 or so compounds in the plant which are structurally related to THC are collectively called cannabinoids.

THC was detected in the breast milk of two women who smoked cannabis every day.[41] One woman smoked cannabis once daily the other seven times per day. In the latter case the milk:plasma ratio of THC concentrations was 8:1. THC and its metabolites were detected in this infant's faeces suggesting that THC had been absorbed and metabolised. Despite this, neither of the infants appeared to suffer any adverse effects.

Twenty-seven infants whose mothers had smoked cannabis during lactation were assessed at one year of age.[42] There were no differences between exposed infants and 35 controls in terms of stature, age at weaning, and mental and motor development. By contrast, an investigation of 68 infants exposed to cannabis via breast milk revealed an association with decreased motor development at one year of age, compared to an equal number of matched controls.[43]

THC enters breast milk and may accumulate. In adults, a single dose of cannabis can take up to a month to be eliminated from the body, since cannabinoids partition into fatty tissues from which they are slowly released. Acute adverse effects upon the breast-fed infant have not been described and the long-term effects are unclear – therefore, mothers should not use cannabis and breastfeed.

Cocaine

Pregnancy

The effects of cocaine upon human pregnancy outcome have been more extensively studied than those of any other street drug. Cocaine causes vasoconstriction and increased blood pressure. This might be expected to increase the risk of spontaneous abortion, abruptio placentae, prematurity, low birth weight and sudden labour. A large number of studies have confirmed that cocaine use in pregnancy is associated with increased risk of all five complications.[33,44–47] However, there is a complex link between these outcomes and duration/extent of cocaine use, lifestyle, demography, access to healthcare facilities and use of other substances. For example, providing prenatal care facilities to cocaine users seems to reduce dramatically the incidence of low birth weight, prematurity and abruptio placentae, or eliminates the risk entirely.[48–52] Unfortunately, a large proportion of the other published studies do not control adequately for this and other confounding variables, and the details of cocaine use in pregnancy are often sketchy. It is true to say that cocaine use is associated with an increased risk of abortion, abruption, prematurity, low birth weight and precipitate labour, but the extent of cocaine's direct pharmacological role in these events is still uncertain. At one extreme, cocaine could simply be a marker for other more important determinants.

There are roughly equal numbers of studies, of small to intermediate size, showing that cocaine does increase or does not increase the overall incidence of fetal abnormalities. Those that show an increased incidence do not generally reveal a particular pattern to these events. However, some investigations have suggested a link to specific organ damage and these are discussed below.

Some studies suggest that cocaine can cause vascular-mediated brain damage in the fetus, in the same way as in adults. In one of the earliest studies of its kind, 13 of 32 cocaine-exposed neonates examined by cranial ultrasound were found to have brain anomalies suggestive of CNS vascular damage.[53] Another study reported that the frequency of abnormal CNS ultrasound findings was the same in cocaine-exposed and non-exposed neonates. However, when the same data were re-analysed and cocaine users were divided into light and heavy users, the frequency of ultrasound defects was greater in the heavy cocaine users.[54] Brain lesions may be the result of *in utero* haemorrhage, ischaemia or infarction, all of which are known to occur in adults who abuse the drug. Other small studies and case reports have actually described clinical brain damage that appeared to have a vascular basis.[55–57] A study of 16 cocaine-exposed neonates with convulsions revealed one to have a brain infarct and six of the babies continued to suffer from convulsions six months later.[58]

Several studies suggest that cocaine use might be associated with fetal urinary and/or genital defects. For example, one study of 52 long-term cocaine users revealed nine infants with genitourinary defects.[59] Studies of a similar size that do not reveal a link have been reported; a major study of 1324 cocaine-exposed children found no increased incidence of urogenital anomalies of any kind.[60]

Other papers have suggested an association between cocaine use in pregnancy and the following fetal anomalies: necrotising enterocolitis,[61] auditory system defects,[62] congenital heart disease,[63] and limb defects.[64] However, the data to support these associations are much weaker than that for CNS or urogenital defects.

Several studies have associated *in utero* cocaine exposure with an increased risk of sudden infant death syndrome (SIDS).[65–68] Cocaine may be a marker for some other cause and a direct causative role would be difficult to prove. However, a possible aetiological mechanism exists, since cocaine exposure in pregnancy has been associated with abnormal respiratory patterns in infants (e.g. increased respiratory pauses, episodes of apnoea and abnormal breathing patterns).[69,70]

Neurobehavioural studies of cocaine-exposed infants have yielded conflicting results and no consensus has yet been reached. Later development can clearly be prejudiced by any cognitive or behavioural changes wrought by cocaine, together with its physical effects.

Breastfeeding

Cocaine does not seem to affect human prolactin levels and so would not be expected to affect the breastfeeding process. However, three case reports describe the passage of the drug into human milk.

- The first case described the repeated nasal inhalation of cocaine by a breastfeeding mother.[71] During a four-hour period approximately 0.5 g was used and the 14-day old baby was fed from the breast five times. The baby developed several adverse effects including irritability, vomiting, diarrhoea, mydriasis, tachycardia, tachypnoea, hypertension and tremor. A range of reflexes were also accentuated and symptoms did not resolve completely for 60 hours. The baby's urine contained cocaine and its metabolites for five consecutive analyses over a 48-hour period, but was negative at 60 hours.

- In the second documented case, analysis of breast milk from a woman known to use cocaine, revealed the drug and its metabolites in her milk.[72] The neonate was noted to be persistently agitated and it was suspected that the mother breast-fed. Unfortunately, neither the urine nor blood of the baby was analysed. The authors speculated that unionised cocaine would become trapped in breast milk (which is more acidic than plasma) and that passage into milk would be further facilitated by the lipophilic nature of the drug. They estimated that cocaine could reach very high concentrations in human milk, and could exceed maternal plasma concentration by a factor of 20 or more.
- A third report described a breast-fed baby whose mother used cocaine.[73] His urine contained cocaine, but no mention is made of any ill effects.

In view of these three cases, women should not take cocaine and breastfeed since the drug can clearly pass into breast milk and may be concentrated there. Cocaine in breast milk is well absorbed from the infant's gut. Furthermore, neonates are deficient in the plasma esterase enzymes which metabolise cocaine and so the drug may accumulate and/or have prolonged adverse effects (as in the first case above).

LSD

Pregnancy

Of all the major drugs of abuse, LSD has been studied the least. The medical literature contains several case reports of congenitally deformed babies born to women who abused LSD, but there is no consistent pattern to these effects and their relevance is unknown. There is an inherent reporting bias, since adverse pregnancy outcomes are much more likely to be documented than uneventful ones. Case reports often fail to describe maternal use of other substances, obstetric history and the trimester(s) of exposure, and rely on maternal recall to assess LSD use.

In 1972, a team of researchers followed 138 pregnancies in women who were known to use LSD and other street drugs.[74] Only 58 women actually took LSD during pregnancy, but the frequency of use, dose and trimester of exposure are not given. Three of these women were delivered of malformed babies – two had confined LSD use to the first trimester only, and the other one had used LSD in both the second and third trimesters. One of the first trimester users had also used a wide range of other street drugs, the others had not. All of the remaining 55 pregnancies where LSD was taken, ended in either normal healthy babies or abortion (spontaneous or therapeutic). Unfortunately, because of the method of data presentation it is not possible to differentiate between these. None of the normal infants were underweight or undersized. Forty-three per cent of the women recruited before the 12th week of pregnancy are stated to have suffered a spontaneous abortion. Regrettably, it is not documented whether these women even took LSD in pregnancy.

Another apparently large study has serious flaws. A follow-up of 121 pregnancies, where parental use of LSD was known from medical records, revealed that only 12 pregnancies involved the use of LSD during pregnancy.[75] Of these, six were in the same woman (five spontaneous abortions and one normal infant). Of the remaining six, one pregnancy ended in spontaneous abortion, the other five were presumably normal.

In a series of 10 children, eight of whom were exposed to LSD in the first trimester, all babies were normal, but three were born prematurely.[76] In 1971, Dumars reported on 47 babies whose parents were known to have used LSD, but not necessarily during pregnancy.[77] Twenty-one of the women had used LSD during pregnancy – at least 19 of them in the first trimester. From the total of 47 women involved, six different neonatal abnormalities were described; two further neonates suffered from convulsions. It is not clear whether these eight babies were exposed to LSD *in utero* or not. Many of the mothers had used a wide range of other drugs in addition to LSD during pregnancy. Smoking and alcohol intake was not assessed. It is assumed that the remaining 39 babies were all normal, although this is not actually stated.

In summary, the data concerning LSD use in human pregnancy are of poor quality. Although many reviewers have come to the conclusion that LSD is not teratogenic, the published data are insufficient to confirm this optimism and further study is needed.

Breastfeeding

There are no studies or case reports of LSD use during human lactation, and it is not known whether the drug penetrates into human milk. Consequently, LSD should not be taken during breastfeeding because it has potent psychedelic effects even at very low dosage and the potential effects upon the suckling infant are impossible to predict.

In non-lactating rats, LSD reduces the secretion of prolactin.[78,79] If this occurred in breastfeeding women, there might be reduced milk flow. However, permanent impairment of milk flow is only likely when prolonged inhibition of prolactin secretion occurs, and most LSD users tend not to take the drug every day. The half-life of LSD is approximately eight hours.

Opioids

Pregnancy

A large number of studies have revealed the effects of heroin (diamorphine) abuse and methadone maintenance on the outcome of human pregnancy. Several reviews have been written, the main findings of which are as follows.[80–83]

- Opioids are not associated with an increased risk of fetal malformations.
- The incidence of spontaneous abortion is not increased.
- Intra-uterine growth retardation is a common finding in most studies, manifested as reduced birth weight, length and head size. The relative contribution of direct opioid effects and maternal lifestyle have not been clearly delineated. The effect can persist into childhood.
- There is evidence that maternal heroin or methadone use is associated with prematurity.
- Neonatal opioid withdrawal is very common. It is probably a dose-related phenomenon, being both more likely and more severe as the dose of opioid increases. At maternal doses less than 20 mg methadone per day, neonatal withdrawal is less common. Symptoms typically develop within 48 hours of birth for heroin-dependent neonates and within seven days for the methadone dependent (*see* Box 18.1). Symptoms are less severe and of a shorter duration with heroin, compared to methadone. Occasionally, methadone withdrawal may take two weeks or more to manifest. Heroin withdrawal is usually less prolonged than that caused by methadone. Sub-acute withdrawal symptoms, consisting of hyperactivity and behavioural problems, may persist for months in some infants.
- SIDS is more common in babies exposed to opioids during pregnancy.
- Small behavioural and intellectual deficits have been identified in some children exposed to heroin or methadone *in utero*. Other studies have shown no adverse effects. It is difficult to differentiate between a drug as the cause, or the social/health problems which tend to be associated with the children of substance misusers. It is also unclear whether any of these changes are important or permanent.

Box 18.1:   Signs and symptoms of opioid withdrawal in the neonate

- Hypertonia, twitching, hyperactive Moro reflex, tremor, convulsions.
- Sleeplessness, restlessness, agitation, irritability, scratching.
- Tachypnoea, high-pitched cry, yawning, sneezing, snuffling, respiratory alkalosis.
- Diarrhoea and vomiting.
- Poor feeding, excessive suck, weight loss, failure to gain weight.
- Hypertension, tachycardia.
- Temperature instability.
- Lacrimation.

Breastfeeding

All opioids pass into breast milk in measurable quantities but for individual opioids the published data are limited. There are no recent data on diamorphine (heroin) although many reviews cite references from 1915–1940 as evidence of diamorphine passage into human breast milk; these papers are of no scientific value.[84,85] Collectively they contend that diamorphine use by the mother can ameliorate symptoms of neonatal opioid withdrawal, or can cause symptoms of intoxication in the neonate. They cannot be relied upon.

Methadone is the most extensively studied opioid. One case report suggested that methadone delivered to an infant via breast milk could have been responsible for its death – however, it also suggested that maternal poisoning of the infant by administration of oral methadone was also a very real possibility.[86] In addition, the infant had multiple pre-existing organ damage and at autopsy had a plasma methadone level which was not high by adult standards. Apart from this case report, the published studies seem to show that at the normal doses used to prevent opioid withdrawal, the amount of methadone in breast milk is unlikely to pose a risk to the suckling infant. Compared to other opioids, methadone is highly bound to plasma proteins and tissues. This attribute limits the extent to which the drug may pass into breast milk. Methadone does not concentrate in breast milk and is found in lower concentrations in milk than in maternal plasma. The American Academy of Pediatrics[87] suggests that the maximum dose to be taken by breastfeeding mothers should be 20 mg daily, but this dose is quite arbitrary and not based on any published studies.

Since diamorphine is converted to morphine, one can consider these two opioids together. The limited information suggests that morphine does not penetrate breast milk in very large amounts. Rivers reported that mothers who take large doses of intravenous heroin are frequently physically unable to breastfeed,[88] but offered no published research or explanation to support this.

Pethidine and its major metabolite norpethidine appear to concentrate in breast milk. Even short-term administration has been shown to have adverse neurobehavioural effects upon breast-fed infants, compared to recipients of morphine.[89] For this reason it should be avoided.

In summary, data on opioid passage into human milk is fragmentary. The available evidence suggests that methadone, morphine and diamorphine are not likely to enter breast milk in sufficient quantities to cause harm to the infant, unless the mother is taking exceptionally large doses. Nevertheless, opioids are metabolised very slowly in infants, so there is a risk of accumulation with prolonged exposure. Mothers should be aware of this possibility and seek medical assistance in the event of any unusual infant sedation. Mothers should breastfeed immediately before an opioid dose is taken to avoid peak concentrations of opioid in milk. Regular pethidine use should be avoided by breastfeeding women.

Volatile substance abuse (VSA)

Pregnancy

It is very difficult to give advice about the potential harm to the fetus of solvent abuse during pregnancy. With the exception of toluene, most of the published data are derived from occupational exposure to specific solvents which involves a much lower level of exposure than that encountered by chronic solvent abusers.

Several epidemiological studies have suggested that women who work in solvent-laden environments are more likely to suffer from miscarriage.[90–92] However, the results of at least two of these studies are not statistically significant when patients' gravidity is accounted for.[90,92] In another study only certain classes of solvents appeared to have an adverse effect which was often inconsistent (e.g. paradoxically occurring at low doses but not at higher doses).[93] Other studies have not shown a link between solvent exposure and increased risk of miscarriage.[94–96]

Individual studies of occupational exposure to various solvents in pregnancy have suggested links to the following neonatal anomalies:

*   general increased risk of malformations
*   CNS defects
*   oesophageal stenosis or atresia
*   omphalocele or gastroschisis
*   cardiovascular damage
*   cleft palate.

However, in all these epidemiological studies it is impossible to account for all potentially confounding variables.

There has been particular interest in the effects of toluene abuse upon human pregnancy outcome. Four studies reported the effects of chronic toluene exposure during pregnancy on a total of 77 neonates.[97–100] Collectively they show that about 40% of exposed babies were born prematurely, and that 50% were of low birth weight for gestational age. In addition, approximately one-third suffered from microcephaly and 9% across the four studies died in the perinatal period. The authors noted the existence of minor craniofacial anomalies in many infants. This dysmorphism has led some to suggest that sufferers may be experiencing 'fetal toluene syndrome' or 'fetal solvent syndrome'. Classic features which have been described include:

- small jaw
- shortened palpebral fissures
- ear anomalies (structural not functional)
- small mid-face
- flattened nose bridge
- a narrow bifrontal diameter
- smooth philtrum
- thin upper lip
- small nose
- abnormal cranial hair pattern.

Within the four studies only 29 babies were formally examined for evidence of facial dysmorphism, but 26 of these exhibited some degree of dysmorphism.

In two studies, a proportion of infants was developmentally assessed at about one year of age. Arnold *et al.* found cognitive or motor delay in nine of 24 infants, and speech delay in nine of 24.[100] Eleven were underweight, nine were below average height and 11 suffered from microcephaly. Similarly, Wilkins-Haug and Gabow reported some measure of growth retardation in eight of 13 exposed infants, and microcephaly in seven.[98]

Toluene abuse in pregnancy has also been associated with maternal renal tubular acidosis, which was first described by Goodwin in five women.[101] Three of these were delivered of babies that were small for gestational age; two had craniofacial anomalies and two developed neonatal acidosis. Acidosis developed in 14 of the pregnancies described by Wilkins-Haug and Gabow,[98] and in five of those described by Pearson *et al.*[99] The fetus is likely to be at greatest risk of harm when the mother actually experiences solvent toxicity whilst pregnant.

Finally, one study has suggested that maternal VSA during pregnancy can be associated with a withdrawal reaction in the neonate.[102] Typical signs described in the newborn were excessive crying, high-pitched cry, sleeplessness, tremulousness, hypotonia, and poor feeding. Of 48 babies born to mothers who engaged in VSA, 32 showed symptoms severe enough to be treated. In the event, only 27 of these received pharmacotherapy (with phenobarbitone) which was judged effective in 17.

Breastfeeding

It is not known whether volatile substances will cross into breast milk or harm the infant. However, the volatile substances that are subject to abuse are very small lipophilic molecules, so passage into breast milk seems inevitable. Fortunately, this group of substances is excreted from the body very rapidly, so it is unlikely that the infant would be exposed to a significant dose of the substance unless the mother breast-fed while actually intoxicated. Even in this situation it is not clear whether volatile substances would be absorbed from the baby's gastrointestinal tract.

Table 18.1: Summary table

Drug	Effects on fetus	Neonatal withdrawal reported
Amphetamine (and Ecstasy)	• Prematurity, reduced growth and microcephaly, but unclear that drug is directly responsible. • Ecstasy may significantly increase the risk of cardiovascular and musculoskeletal anomalies.	+
Anabolic steroids	• Decreased maternal fertility. • Virilisation of female fetuses.	–
Cannabis	• Tenuous link to delayed infant CNS maturation, but unproven. • Weak link to childhood cancer, but not proven. • Probably does not cause malformations.	–
Cocaine	• Increased risk of reduced growth, spontaneous abortion, prematurity and abruption, but unclear that drug is directly responsible. • Vascular brain damage can occur, but is rare. • Insufficient evidence that drug can cause other malformations. • Possibly linked to SIDS.	–
LSD	• Insufficient information.	–
Opioids (heroin and methadone)	• Reduced growth and prematurity, but unclear whether the drugs are directly responsible. • Probably do not cause malformations. • Possibly linked to SIDS.	+++
Volatile substances	• Weak link to facial dysmorphism, but more study needed for confirmation. • Possible increased risk of spontaneous abortion, low birth weight and prematurity, but direct role of volatile substances is unclear.	+

References

1 Nora JJ, Vargo TA, Nora AH *et al.* (1970) Dexamphetamine: a possible environmental trigger in cardiovascular malformations. *Lancet.* **I**: 1290.

2 McElhatton PR, Bateman DN, Evans C *et al.* (1998) Does exposure to 'amphetamine' in pregnancy cause congenital malformations? A prospective follow-up of 129 pregnancies. *UK Drug Information Conference Proceedings.* **5**: 67.

3 Nora JJ, McNamara DG and Fraser FC (1967) Dexamphetamine sulphate and human malformations. *Lancet.* **I**: 570–1.

4 Milkovich L and van den Berg BJ (1977) Effects of antenatal exposure to anorectic drugs. *Am J Obs Gynecol.* **129**: 637–42.

5 Little BB, Snell LM and Gilstrap LC (1988) Methamphetamine abuse during pregnancy: outcome and fetal effects. *Obs Gynecol.* **72**: 541–4.

6 Heinonen OP, Slone D and Shapiro S (1977) *Birth Defects and Drugs in Pregnancy.* Publishing Sciences Group, Littleton.

7 Levin JN (1971) Amphetamine ingestion with biliary atresia. *J Pediatr.* **79**: 130–1.

8 Oro AS and Dixon SD (1987) Perinatal cocaine and methamphetamine exposure: maternal and neonatal correlates. *J Pediatr.* **111**: 571–8.

9 Gillogley K, Evans A, Hansen R *et al.* (1990) The perinatal impact of cocaine, amphetamine and opiate use detected by universal intra-partum screening. *Am J Obs Gynecol.* **163**: 1535–42.

10 Eriksson M, Larsson G *et al.* (1978) The influence of amphetamine addiction on pregnancy and the newborn infant. *Acta Paed Scand.* **67**: 95–9.

11 Dixon SD (1989) Effects of transplacental exposure to cocaine and methamphetamine on the neonate. *West J Med.* **150**: 436–42.

12 Eriksson M and Zetterstrom R (1994) Amphetamine addiction during pregnancy: 10 year follow-up. *Acta Paed Scand.* **83**: 27–31.

13 Eriksson M, Jonsson B, Steneroth G and Zetterstrom R (1994) Cross-sectional growth of children whose mothers abused amphetamines during pregnancy. *Acta Paed Scand.* **83**: 612–17.

14 Green AR and Goodwin GM (1996) Ecstasy and neurodegeneration. *BMJ.* **312**: 1493–4.

15 Steiner E, Villen T, Hallberg M and Rane A (1984) Amphetamine secretion in breast milk. *Eur J Clin Pharmacol.* **27**: 123–4.

16 Ayd F (1973) Excretion of psychotropic drugs in human breast milk. *International Drug Therapy Newsletter.* **8**: 33–40.

17 DeLeo V, Cella SG, Camanni F *et al.* (1983) Prolactin lowering effect of amphetamine in normoprolactinemic subjects and in physiological and pathological hyperprolactinemia. *Hormone Metabolic Res.* **15**: 439–43.

18 Petraglia F, DeLeo V, Sardelli S *et al.* (1987) Prolactin changes after administration of agonist and antagonist dopaminergic drugs in puerperal women. *Gynecol Obs Invest.* **23**: 103–9.

19 Grumbach MM and Ducharme JR (1960) The effects of androgens on fetal sexual development. *Fertil Steri.* **11**: 157–80.

20 Rosa, FW (1984) Virilisation of the female fetus with maternal danazol exposure. *Am J Obs Gynecol.* **149**: 99–100.

21 Shaw RW and Farquhar JW (1984) Female pseudohermaphroditism associated with danazol exposure *in utero*. Case report. *Br J Obs Gynecol.* **91**: 386–9.

22 Duck SC and Katayama KP (1981) Danazol may cause female pseudohermaphroditism. *Fertil Steril.* **35**: 230–1.

23 Peress MR, Kreutner AK, Mathur RS and Williamson HO (1982) Female pseudohermaphroditism with somatic chromosomal anomaly in association with *in utero* exposure to danazol. *Am J Obs Gynecol.* **142**: 708–9.

24 Castro-Magana M, Cheruvanky T, Collipp PJ *et al.* (1981) Transient adrenogenital syndrome due to exposure to danazol *in utero*. *Am J Dis Child.* **135**: 1032–4.

25 Money J and Mathews D (1982) Prenatal exposure to virilising progestins: an adult follow-up study of twelve women. *Arch Sex Behav.* **11**: 73–83.

26 Reschini E, Giustina G, D'Alberton A and Candiani GB (1985) Female pseudohermaphroditism due to maternal androgen administration: 25-year follow-up. *Lancet.* **i**: 1226.

27 Dewhurst J and Gordon RR (1984) Fertility following change of sex. *Lancet.* **ii**: 1461.

28 Dodek SM, Friedman JM, Soyster PA and Marcellus HL (1954) Intrapartum initiation of lactation control with a long-acting androgen. *J Am Med Assoc.* **154**: 309–11.

29 Roland M, Veprovsky E, Linhart W *et al.* (1955) The use of various endocrine preparations in the suppression of lactation: a comparative study in 800 cases. *Am J Obstet Gynecol.* **70**: 1004–11.

30 Lass PM (1942) The inhibition of lactation during the puerperium by methyl testosterone. *Am J Obstet Gynecol.* **43**: 86–93.

31 Biggs JSG, Hacker N and Andrews E (1978) Bromocriptine, methyltestosterone and placebo for inhibition of physiological lactation. *Med J Aust.* **2**(4): 23–5.

32 Gold JJ, Soihet S, Hankin H and Cohen MR (1959) Hormone therapy to control postpartum breast manifestations. *Am J Obstet Gynecol.* **78**: 86–95.

33 Richardson GA, Day NL and McGauhey PJ (1993) The impact of prenatal marijuana and cocaine use on the infant and child. *Clin Obstet Gynecol.* **36**: 302–18.

34 Marijuana (1994) In: GG Briggs, RK Freeman and SJ Yaffe (eds) *Drugs in Pregnancy and Lactation*. Williams & Wilkins, Baltimore, pp. 519–30.

35 Marijuana (1994) In: JM Friedman and JE Polifka (eds) *Teratogenic Effects of Drugs: a resource for clinicians*. Johns Hopkins, Baltimore.

36 Cannabis (1990) In: PI Folb and MNG Dukes (eds) *Drug Safety in Pregnancy*. Elsevier, Amsterdam, pp. 53–6.

37 Fried PA (1993) Prenatal exposure to tobacco and marijuana: effects during pregnancy, infancy and early childhood. *Clin Obstet Gynecol.* **36**: 319–37.

38 Hingson R, Alpert JJ, Day N *et al.* (1982) Effects of maternal drinking and marijuana use on fetal growth and development. *Pediatrics.* **70**: 539–46.

39 Robison LL, Buckley JD, Daigle AE *et al.* (1989) Maternal drug use and risk of childhood non-lymphoblastic leukaemia among offspring: an epidemiologic investigation implicating marijuana. *Cancer.* **63**: 1904–11.

40 Grufferman S, Schwartz AG, Ruymann B and Maurer HM (1993) Parents' use of cocaine and marijuana and increased risk of rhabdomyosarcoma in their children. *Cancer Causes Control.* **4**: 217–24.

41 Peres-Reges M and Wall ME (1982) Presence of tetrahydrocannabinol in human milk, *New Engl J Med.* **307**: 819–20.

42 Tennes K, Avitable N, Blackard C *et al.* (1985) Marijuana: prenatal and postnatal exposure in the human. *NIDA Res Mono.* **59**: 48–60.

43 Astley SJ and Little RE (1990) Maternal marijuana use during lactation and infant development at one year. *Neurotoxicol Teratol.* **12**: 161–8.

44   Volpe JJ (1992) Effect of cocaine use on the fetus. *New Engl J Med.* **327**: 399–407.

45   Zuckerman B, Frank D and Brown E (1995) Overview of the effects of abuse and drugs on pregnancy and offspring. In: Medications development for the treatment of pregnant addicts and their infants. *NIDA Res Mono.* **149**: 16–38.

46   Cocaine (1994) In: GG Briggs, RK Freeman and SJ Yaffe (eds) *Drugs in Pregnancy and Lactation.* Williams & Wilkins, Baltimore, pp. 200–16.

47   Cocaine (1990) In: PI Folb and MNG Dukes (eds) *Drug Safety in Pregnancy.* Elsevier, Amsterdam, pp. 56–9.

48   Chazotte C, Youchah J and Freda MC (1995) Cocaine use during pregnancy and low birth weight: the impact of prenatal care and drug treatment, *Seminars Perinatol.* **19**: 293–300.

49   Miller Jr JM, Boudreaux MC and Regan FA (1995) A case–control study of cocaine use in pregnancy. *Am J Obs Gynecol.* **172**: 180–5.

50   MacGregor SN, Keith LG, Bachicha JA and Chasnoff IJ (1989) Cocaine abuse during pregnancy: correlation between prenatal care and perinatal outcome. *Obstet Gynecol.* **74**: 882.

51   Zuckerman BS, Frank D, Hingson R *et al.* (1989) Effects of maternal marijuana and cocaine use on fetal growth. *New Engl J Med.* **320**: 762–8.

52   Shiono PH, Klebanoff MA, Nugent RP *et al.* (1995) The impact of cocaine and marijuana use on low birth weight and preterm birth: a multicenter study. *Am J Obs Gynecol.* **172**: 19–27.

53   Dixon SD and Bejar R (1989) Echoencephalographic findings in neonates associated with maternal cocaine and methamphetamine use: incidence and clinical correlates. *J Pediatrics.* **115**: 770–8.

54   Frank D, McKarten K, Cabral H *et al.* (1994) Association of heavy *in utero* cocaine exposure with caudate haemorrhage in term newborns. *Pediatr Res.* **35**: 269A.

55   Chasnoff IJ, Bussey ME and Savich R (1987) Perinatal cerebral infarction and maternal cocaine use. *J Pediatr.* **111**: 571–8.

56   Kapur RP, Shaw CM and Shepard TH (1991) Brain haemorrhages in cocaine-exposed human fetuses. *Teratology.* **44**: 11–18.

57   Dominguez R, Vila-Coro AA, Slopis JM *et al.* (1991) Brain and ocular abnormalities in infants with *in utero* exposure to cocaine and other street drugs. *Am J Dis Child.* **145**: 688–95.

58   Kramer LD, Locke GE and Ogunyemi A (1990) Neonatal cocaine-related seizures. *J Child Neurol.* **5**: 60–4.

59   Chasnoff IJ, Chisum GM and Kaplan WE (1988) Maternal cocaine use and genitourinary tract malformations. *Teratology.* **37**: 201–4.

60   Rajegowda B, Lala R, Nagaraj A *et al.* (1991) Does cocaine increase congenital urogenital abnormalities in newborns? *Pediatr Res.* **29**: 71A.

61   Porat R and Brodsky N (1991) Cocaine: a risk factor for necrotizing enterocolitis. *J Perinatol.* **11**: 30–2.

62   Shih L, Cone-Wesson B and Reddix B (1988) Effects of maternal cocaine abuse on the neonatal auditory system. *Int J Pediatr Otorhinolaryngol.* **15**: 245–51.

63   Lipschultz SE, Frassica JJ and Orav EJ (1991) Cardiovascular abnormalities in infants prenatally exposed to cocaine. *J Pediatr.* **118**: 44–51.

64   Hoyme HE, Jones KL and Dixon SD (1990) Prenatal cocaine exposure and fetal vascular disruption. *Pediatrics.* **85**: 743–7.

65   Durand DJ, Espinoza AM and Nickerson BJ (1990) Association between prenatal cocaine exposure and sudden infant death syndrome. *J Pediatr.* **117**: 909–11.

66 Chasnoff IJ, Burns KA and Burns WJ (1987) Cocaine use in pregnancy: perinatal mortality and morbidity. *Neurotoxicol Teratol.* **9**: 291–3.

67 Kandall SR, Gaines J, Davidson D and Jessop G (1993) Relationship of maternal substance abuse to subsequent sudden infant death syndrome in offspring. *J Pediatr.* **123**: 120–6.

68 Bauchner H, Zuckerman B, McClain M *et al.* (1988) Risk of sudden infant death syndrome among infants with *in utero* exposure to cocaine. *J Pediatr.* **113**: 831–4.

69 Chen C, Duara S, Neto GS *et al.* (1991) Clinical and laboratory observations: respiratory instability in neonates with *in utero* exposure to cocaine. *J Pediatr.* **119**: 111–13.

70 Chasnoff IJ, Hunt CE, Kletter R and Kaplan D (1989) Prenatal cocaine exposure is associated with respiratory pattern abnormalities. *Am J Dis Child.* **143**: 583–7.

71 Chasnoff IJ, Lewis DE and Squires L (1987) Cocaine intoxication in a breast fed infant. *Pediatrics.* **80**: 836–8.

72 Dickson PH, Lind A, Studts P *et al.* (1994) The routine analysis of breast milk for drugs of abuse in a clinical toxicology laboratory. *J Forensic Sci.* **39**: 207–14.

73 Shannon M, Lacouture PG, Roa J and Woolf A (1989) Cocaine exposure among children seen at a pediatric hospital. *Pediatrics.* **83**: 337–42.

74 Jacobson CB and Berlin CM (1972) Possible reproductive detriment in LSD users. *J Am Med Assoc.* **222**: 1367–73.

75 McGlothin WH, Sparkes RS and Arnold DO (1970) Effect of LSD on human pregnancy. *J Am Med Assoc.* **212**: 1483.

76 Aase JM, Laestadius N and Smith DW (1970) Children of mothers who took LSD in pregnancy. *Lancet.* **2**: 100–1.

77 Dumars KW (1971) Parental drug usage: effect upon chromosomes of progeny. *Pediatrics.* **47**: 1037–41.

78 Meltzer HY, Fesler RG, Simonovic M *et al.* (1977) Lysergic acid diethylamide: evidence for stimulation of pituitary dopamine receptors, *Psychopharmacol.* **54**: 39–44.

79 Horowski R and Graf KJ (1979) Neuroendocrine effects of neuropsychotropic drugs and their possible influence on toxic reactions in animals and man – the role of the dopamine-prolactin system. *Archiv Toxicol.* **2**(1): 93–104.

80 Jarvis MAE and Schnoll SH (1995) Methadone use during pregnancy. In: Medications development for the treatment of pregnant addicts and their infants. *NIDA Res Mon.* **149**: 58–77.

81 Hoegerman G and Schnoll S (1991) Narcotic use in pregnancy. *Clin Perinatol.* **18**: 51–76.

82 Rosen TS and Johnson HL (1993) Prenatal methadone maintenance: its effects on fetus, neonate and child. *Dev Brain Dysfunct.* **6**: 317–23.

83 Heroin and methadone (1994) In: GG Briggs, RK Freeman and SJ Yaffe (eds) *Drugs in Pregnancy and Lactation.* Williams & Wilkins, Baltimore, pp. 413–15 and 556–8.

84 Cobrinik RW, Hood RT and Chusid E (1959) The effect of maternal narcotic addiction on the newborn infant. *Pediatrics.* **24**: 288–304.

85 Lichtenstein PM (1915) Infant drug addicts. *NY Med J.* **102**: 905.

86 Smialek JE, Monforte JR, Aronow R *et al.* (1977) Methadone deaths in children: a continuing problem. *J Am Med Assoc.* **238**: 2516–57.

87 Committee on Drugs (1994) The transfer of drugs and other chemicals into human milk. *Pediatrics.* **93**: 137–50.

88 Rivers RPA (1986) Neonatal opiate withdrawal. *Arch Dis Child.* **61**: 1236–9.

89 Wittels MD, Scott DT and Sinatra RS (1990) Exogenous opioids in human breast milk and acute neonatal behavior: a preliminary study. *Anesthesiol.* **73**: 864–9.

90 Strandberg M, Sandback K, Axelson O and Sundell L (1978) Spontaneous abortion in women in hospital laboratory. *Lancet.* **i**: 384–5.

91 Lindbohm M-L, Taskinen H, Sallmen M and Hemminki K (1990) Spontaneous abortions among women exposed to organic solvents. *Am J Industrial Med.* **17**: 449–63.

92 Heidan LZ (1983) Spontaneous abortions among factory workers. The importance of gravidity control. *Scand J Soc Med.* **11**: 81–5.

93 Windham GC, Shusterman D, Swan SH *et al.* (1991) Exposure to organic solvents and adverse pregnancy outcome. *Am J Industrial Med.* **20**: 241–59.

94 Ahlborg Jr G (1990) Pregnancy outcome among women working in laundries and dry-cleaning shops using tetrachloroethylene. *Am J Industrial Med.* **17**: 567–75.

95 Mur JM, Mandereau L, Deplan F *et al.* (1992) Spontaneous abortion and exposure to vinyl chloride. *Lancet.* **339**: 127–8.

96 Axelson G, Liutz C and Rylander R (1984) Exposure to solvents and outcome of pregnancy in university laboratory employees. *Br J Industrial Med.* **41**: 305–12.

97 Hersh JH, Podruch PE, Rogers G and Weisskopf B (1985) Toluene embryopathy. *J Pediatrics.* **106**: 922–7.

98 Wilkins-Haug L and Gabow PA (1991) Toluene abuse during pregnancy: obstetric complications and perinatal outcomes. *Obstet Gynecol.* **77**: 504–9.

99 Pearson MA, Hoyme HE, Seaver LH and Rimsza ME (1994) Toluene embryopathy: delineation of the phenotype and comparison with fetal alcohol syndrome. *Pediatrics.* **93**: 211–15.

100 Arnold GL, Kirby RS, Langendoerfer S and Wilkins-Haug L (1994) Toluene embryopathy: clinical delineation and developmental follow-up. *Pediatrics.* **93**: 216–20.

101 Goodwin TH (1988) Toluene abuse and renal tubular acidosis in pregnancy. *Obstet Gynecol.* **71**: 715–18.

102 Tenebein M, Casiro OG, Seshia MMK and Debooy VD (1996) Neonatal withdrawal from maternal volatile substance abuse. *Arch Dis Child.* **74**: F204–7.

Further reading

Blinick G, Inturrisi CE, Jerez E and Wallach RC (1975) Methadone assays in pregnant women and progeny. *Am J Obs Gyn.* **121**: 617–21.

Blinick G, Jerez E and Wallach RC (1973) Methadone maintenance pregnancy, and progeny. *J Am Med Assoc.* **225**: 477–9.

Borgatta L, Jenny RW, Gruss L *et al.* (1997) Clinical significance of methohexital, meperidine, and diazepam in breast milk. *J Clin Pharmacol.* **37**: 186–92.

Catz C and Guiacoia G (1972) Drugs and breast milk. *Pediatric Clin N Am.* **19**: 151–66.

Feilberg VL, Rosenborg D, Christensen CB and Mogensen JV (1989) Excretion of morphine in human breast milk. *Acta Anaesth Scand.* **33**: 426–8.

Findley JWA, DeAngelis RL, Kearney MF *et al.* (1981) Analgesic drugs in breast milk and plasma. *Clin Pharmacol Ther.* **29**: 625–33.

Geraghty B, Graham EA, Logan B and Weiss EL (1997) Methadone levels in breast milk. *J Hum Lactation.* **13**: 227–30.

Horning MG, Stillwell WG, Nowlin J *et al.* (1975) Identification and quantification of drugs and drug metabolites in human breast milk using GC-MS-COM methods. *Mod Probl Paed.* **15**: 73–9.

Kreek MJ, Schecter A, Gutjahr CL *et al.* (1974) Analyses of methadone and other drugs in maternal and neonatal body fluids: use in evaluation of symptoms in a neonate of mother maintained on methadone. *Am J Drug Alcohol Abuse.* **1**: 409–19.

Kunka RL, Venkataraman R, Stern RM and Ladik CF (1984) Excretion of propoxyphene and norpropoxyphene in breast milk. *Clin Pharmacol Ther.* **35**: 675–80.

Kwit NT and Hatcher RA (1935) Excretion of drugs in milk. *Am J Dis Child.* **49**: 900–4.

Leuschen MP, Wolf J and Raybirn WF (1990) Fentanyl excretion in breast milk. *Clin Pharm.* **9**: 336–7.

Peiker VG, Muller B, Ihn W and Noschel H (1980) Ausscheidung von Pethidin durch die Muttermilch. *Zentralblat fur Gynakologie.* **102**: 537–41.

Pond SM, Kreek MJ, Tong TG *et al.* (1985) Altered methadone pharmacokinetics in methadone-maintained pregnant women. *J Pharmacol Exp Ther.* **233**: 1–6.

Rivers RPA (1986) Neonatal opiate withdrawal. *Arch Dis Child.* **61**: 1236–9.

Robieux I, Koren G, Vandenbergh H and Schneiderman J (1990) Morphine excretion in breast milk and resultant exposure of a nursing infant. *Clin Toxicol.* **28**: 365–70.

Smith JW (1982) Codeine-induced bradycardia in a breast-fed infant. *Clin Res.* **30**: 259A.

Wojnar-Horton RE, Kristensen JH, Yapp P *et al.* (1997) Methadone distribution and excretion into breast milk of clients in a methadone maintenance programme. *Br J Clin Pharmacol.* **44**: 543–7.

Index